Instructor's Resource Manual and Test Bank

to accompany

UNDERSTANDING PATHOPHYSIOLOGY

Second Edition

Sue E. Huether, RN, PhD
Kathryn L. McCance, RN, PhD

Prepared by

Kathleen Miller Baldwin, RN, PhD, CEN, CCRN

Associate Professor
Harris College of Nursing
Texas Christian University
Fort Worth, Texas

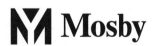

St. Louis Baltimore Boston
Carlsbad Chicago Naples New York Philadelphia Portland
London Madrid Mexico City Singapore Sydney Tokyo Toronto Wiesbaden

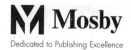

Mosby
Dedicated to Publishing Excellence

Vice President and Nursing Editorial Director: Sally Schrefer
Senior Developmental Editor: Michele D. Hayden
Project Manager: Gayle May Morris
Cover Art: William B. Westwood

Second Edition
Copyright © 2000 by Mosby, Inc.

Mosby, Inc.
A Harcourt Health Sciences Company
11830 Westline Industrial Drive
St. Louis, Missouri 63146

Printed in the United States of America

International Standard Book Number 0-323-00793-7

99 00 01 02 03 WB/EB   9 8 7 6 5 4 3 2 1

www.mosby.com

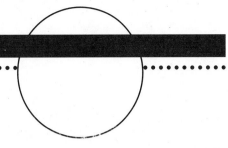

Reviewers

Linda S. Christensen, RN, MSN, JD
Dean of Nursing
Clarkson College
Omaha, Nebraska

Lee A. Farris, RN, MSN
Instructor
Medical College of Georgia–Athens
Athens, Georgia

Sue E. Huether, RN, PhD
Professor, College of Nursing
University of Utah
Salt Lake City, Utah

Marty J. Martin, RN, MSN, FNP
Associate Professor
Jackson Community College
Jackson, Michigan

Registered Nurse
St. Lawrence Hospital
Lansing, Michigan

Kathryn L. McCance, RN, PhD
Professor, College of Nursing
University of Utah
Salt Lake City, Utah

Contents

INSTRUCTOR'S RESOURCE MANUAL

Cellular Biology

OBJECTIVES

After studying this chapter, the learner will be able to:

1. Compare and contrast prokaryotes and eukaryotes.

2. Identify the seven specialized functions of a cell.

3. Discuss the plasma membrane within the framework of the fluid mosaic model, addressing both structural and functional aspects.

4. Identify the three primary methods of cell communication.

5. Define endocrine signaling, paracrine signaling, and synaptic signaling.

6. Describe the process of energy generation and utilization by the cell to support cellular function.

7. Describe the processes of passive transport, diffusion, hydrostatic pressure, and osmosis.

8. Define endocytosis, exocytosis, and mediated active and passive transport, giving examples of each.

9. Discuss the electrochemical changes in the plasma membrane which result in an action potential.

10. Describe cellular reproduction within the four phases of the cell cycle and the four stages of the M phase.

11. Describe how tissues are formed.

12. Name the four basic tissue types.

LECTURE OUTLINE	INSTRUCTOR'S NOTES

Prokaryotes and Eukaryotes
Cellular Functions
Structure and Function of Cellular Components
    Nucleus
    Cytoplasmic organelles
    Cellular receptors
    Plasma membranes
        Membrane composition
    The fluid mosaic model
Cell-to-Cell Communication
Cellular Metabolism
    Role of adenosine triphosphate
    Food and the production of cellular energy
    Oxidative phosphorylationProcesses of Cellular
Intake and Output
    Movement of water and solutes
        Passive transport

LECTURE OUTLINE	**INSTRUCTOR'S NOTES**

          Mediated and active transport
     Transport by vesicle formation
          Endocytosis and exocytosis
          Receptor-mediated endocytosis
     Movement of electrical impulses: membrane
          potentials
Cellular Reproduction: The Cell Cycle
     Phases of mitosis and cytokinesis
     Rates of cellular division
     Growth factors
Tissues
     Tissue formation
     Intercellular communication
     Types of tissues

DIFFICULT CONCEPTS

Cellular Communication

Think of the cell as a "social organizer" producing or directing signals or conversations. Cells communicate with themselves by forming protein channels (gap junctions) for intercellular communication. In certain disease processes like cancer, the cancer cell produces signaling molecules that actually stimulate it to grow, called autocrine stimulation (see Chapter 9). Cells converse with neighbors by producing signals (molecules) that interact with receptors on neighboring cells; this process is called paracrine signaling or intercellular communication. Cells have long distance conversations or extracellular communication by secreting chemicals that signal cells some distances away (endocrine signaling, for example). The analogy of a cell as a "social organizer" can be applied to the movement across the membrane of small, lipid-soluble particles, such as oxygen, carbon dioxide, and urea. Some "messages" take longer to receive than others because substances pass directly through pores, requiring "operator assistance" (transporter molecules expending energy); others require less assistance, with protein transporters moving solutes without expending energy. The analogy of the cell as a social organism helps students understand that injury or disease starts when the conversation breaks down and the cell does not appropriately adapt.

Cellular Metabolism

Cellular matabolism is a term used to describe all chemical functions needed to maintain the cell. Cellular enzymes assist with all of these chemical functions. Cellular metabolism can be further subdivided into anabolism (those processes which need energy to occur) and catabolism (those processes which produce energy when they occur). Energy produced by catabolism is transferred to ATP in the mitochondria. The transfer of energy to ATP is most efficient when oxygen is present (oxidative phosphorylation), but it can occur in the absence of oxygen (anaerobic glycolysis), a less efficient, but reversible process which produces lactic acid. ATP is the cellular molecule which stores energy and delivers it to areas needing it for anabolic cellular processes.

Cellular Reproduction

All body cells except sperm and egg cells reproduce using the processes of mitosis and cytokinesis. Division of the nucleus occurs during mitosis. In cytokinesis the cytoplasm divides after doubling its mass. There are four sequential phases to the cell cycle. Three of the phases, gap 1, synthesis, and gap 2, are often referred to as the interphase. The M phase, where mitosis and cytokinesis occur, is the fourth phase. The gap 1 phase occurs following mitosis, but prior to the onset of synthesis. Before mitosis can occur, additional DNA must be synthesized in the cell nucleus. The period of the cell cycle where this occurs is called the S, or synthesis, phase. This phase is followed by the gap 2 phase, during which RNA and protein synthesis occur. During the M phase, the cell's nuclear membrane disappears, the contents of the nucleus split into two identical halves, the contents of the cytoplasm split into two identical halves, and two cells (daughter cells) are created from the original cell.

CRITICAL THINKING

1. Explain why oxygen (O_2) can easily cross a plasma membrane while sodium ions (Na^+) are unable to cross a plasma membrane.

   Answer: The lipid portion of the plasma membranes is composed of polar or amphipathic lipid molecules. The lipid molecules are arranged with their hydrophilic (water loving) portions at the membrane inner and outer surfaces. The hydrophobic (water hating) portions of the lipid molecule on the inside of the membrane face each other. This creates a "sandwich effect" with a hydrophobic oily core. These components are constructed into a lipid bilayer, forming a selectively permeable barrier. Oxygen is able to easily cross the plasma membrane because it is soluble in lipids. Sodium ions are unable to cross the plasma membrane because they are insoluble in the lipid core of the membrane and, therefore, are actively transported by a pump that uses ATP for energy.

2. Explain cell membrane fluidity.

   Answer: According to the fluid mosaic model, biologic membranes are dynamic and change in response to cell needs. Lipids are very fluid and mobile in the plasma membrane. They not only are asymmetrically distributed but also are capable of fairly free lateral and rotational mobility. Asymmetric distribution of lipids changes plasma fluidity, which affects the flexibility and curvature of membranes. The type of fatty acid and the length of the fatty acid chains affect fluidity. For example, cholesterol, which is a small molecule with small OH head group, occurs at the bilayer surface, decreasing fluidity and increasing the mechanical strength and stability of the membrane. Proteins define the specific function of the membrane because they are asymmetrically distributed. They can be either integral (intrinsic) or peripheral and float either singly or in an aggregate within the membrane. Integral proteins are associated directly with the lipid bilayer. Peripheral membrane proteins are associated ionically with hydrophilic lipid molecule heads or other proteins.

3. Explain why cellular division times vary between different types of cells.

   Answer: The difference between cellular division times is the length of time spent in the G1 phase of the cell cycle. The G_1 phase of the cell cycle is the period of time betweeen the M phase (mitosis) and the start of RNA synthesis (S phase). Although the complete cell cycle lasts 12-24 hours, generally about one hour is required for the four stages of mitosis and cytokinesis. The mechanisms that control cell division depend on social control genes and protein growth factors. When a need arises for new cells, previously non-dividing cells must be triggered rapidly to reenter the cell cycle.

Genes and Genetic Diseases

OBJECTIVES

After review of this chapter, the learner will be able to:

1. Describe the structure and function of DNA.

2. Define the processes of transcription and translation.

3. Describe the normal karyotype.

4. Identify the different mechanisms of mutation.

5. Identify the major chromosomal abnormalities and give examples of each.

6. Differentiate between genotype and phenotype.

7. Describe autosomal dominant, autosomal recessive, and X-linked recessive inheritance modes.

8. Construct a pedigree chart for the occurrence of blue eyes in a family.

9. Describe sex-limited and sex-linked traits and give an example of each.

10. Discuss the process and significance of gene mapping.

11. Discuss the concept of multifactorial inheritance.

LECTURE OUTLINE	INSTRUCTOR'S NOTES

DNA, RNA, and Proteins: Heredity at the Molecular
    Level
    Definitions
        Composition and structure of DNA
        DNA as the genetic code
        Replication of DNA
        Mutation
    From genes to proteins
        Transcription
        Gene splicing
        Translation
Chromosomes
    Chromosome aberrations and associated diseases
        Polyploidy
        Aneuploidy
        Abnormalities of chromosome structure
Elements of Formal Genetics
    Phenotype and genotype
    Dominance and recessiveness
Transmission of Genetic Diseases
    Autosomal dominant inheritance

LECTURE OUTLINE	INSTRUCTOR'S NOTES

DIFFICULT CONCEPTS

Protein Synthesis

The analogy of DNA as a cookbook filled with protein recipes is useful. A temporary working copy of a DNA recipe (gene) is transcribed mRNA, just as a cook might write a recipe on a card to avoid "messing up" the master copy (cookbook). The transcribed recipe (mRNA) is a list of ingredients (amino acids encoded as a "list" of codons) to be assembled in a particular order (just as in cooking, the order of mixing ingredients is often critical). Ribosomes (rRNA) and tRNA are like the countertop or mixing bowl and the measuring scoops—reusable tools needed to assemble the ingredients properly. Like cake recipes in which the batter is prepared according to one recipe and the frosting according to a different recipe, several different polypeptides may be synthesized independently, then later put together as a single quaternary protein. This is analogous to several layers of cake and frosting later being put together to form a single cake.

Genotype versus Phenotype

These two terms need much repetitive usage with examples because their definitions are often confusing for students. Grasping the idea that the environment influences the phenotype is difficult. Using the example of PKU from the textbook can be helpful. Repeating the definition and examples of the concept of penetrance helps students understand the differences between genotype and phenotype.

Transmission of Autosomal Dominant and Recessive Diseases

The 46 chromosomes needed for human reproduction come from the combination of 23 from each parent. Sex is determined from the pairing of two (one from each parent). The other 44 chromosomes form 22 pairs of autosomes that may include autosomal diseases from either parent. Autosomal dominant diseases are rare, and Huntington's disease is the best known example. Characteristics include the following: offspring have a 50% recurrent risk of inheriting the disease, no generation is skipped, and both sexes are equally likely to get the disease. Autosomal recessive diseases are also rare, although there may be many carriers. Cystic fibrosis is the best known example. The disease is seen in children; both sexes are equally likely to be affected; and marriage between relatives may be a factor. If both parents are carriers of the recessive gene, the offspring have a 25% recurrent risk of inheriting the disease and have a 50% chance of being a carrier of the disease. If both parents have the recessive disease, all of their children will have the disease.

Transmission of X-Linked Diseases

X-linked diseases are transmitted by genes located on an X chromosome, which determines sex. The affected X chromosome may come from either parent in female offspring, but it can come from only the mother in male offspring. Characteristics include the following: female offspring are seldom affected; fathers never transmit the disease to sons; affected fathers will pass the trait to all of their daughters, who will become unaffected carriers; and the disease may not be seen in every generation, but the gene will be passed by female carriers. A carrier female will transmit the disease to half her male children and the trait to half her female children, who will then become carriers. If the father is affected and the mother is a carrier, half the female children will have the disease and half will be carriers. Half the male children will have the disease and half will be unaffected. An affected father and a normal mother will produce male offspring without the disease and female offspring who will all be carriers of the disease.

CRITICAL THINKING

1. Explain why XX and XXY somatic cells have Barr bodies and XY somatic cells do not have Barr bodies.

   Answer: An X chromosome codes many gene products and must be present for zygote survival. A Y chromosome does not code many gene products. XX somatic cells (female) and XY somatic cells (male) do not differ in the number of gene products coded by the X chromosome even though females contain two X chromosomes. Apparently only one X chromosome is needed to code most X gene products. Therefore, one of the female X chromosomes is permanently inactivated, resulting in highly condensed intranuclear chromatin bodies called Barr bodies. Males lack Barr bodies because they have only one X chromosome. Males with Klinefelter syndrome (XXY) have Barr bodies because they have two X chromosomes.

2. Why does the loss of chromosome material result in more zygote death than the addition of chromosome material?

   Answer: Deletions and additions of chromosome material result in abnormal chromosome structure, changing DNA templates. This template change ultimately results in the loss of protein synthesis or in abnormal protein synthesis. However, monosomy of any autosome or YO sex chromosomes will always result in zygote death and spontaneous abortion. Deletions of chromosome material cause loss of DNA in a chromosome, resulting in a deficient chromosome that unites with a normal chromosome. Despite having one normal chromosome, some genes and their proteins are lost, resulting in severe physical and mental handicaps. Fetuses with additions of chromosome material have a greater chance of survival. Autosomal trisomies of the thirteenth, eighteenth, or twenty-first chromosomes are seen in live births. Trisomy 21 is seen in 1:800 live births. Sex chromosome aneuploidies are fairly high, occurring in 1:400 males and 1:650 females.

3. Why is it important to isolate and clone disease genes?

   Answer: Once a gene is cllonded, its DNA sequence can be studied to determine the nature and function of the protein encoded by the gene. Cloning gives us the possibility to increase our understanding of the pathophysiology of the disease. It also opens the possibility of creating gene therapy for the disorder.

Altered Cellular and Tissue Biology

OBJECTIVES

After review of this chapter, the learner will be able to:

1. Describe the cellular adaptations made in each of the following processes: atrophy, hypertrophy, hyperplasia, dysplasia, and metaplasia.

2. Discuss specific reasons for each of the above adaptations.

3. Describe the mechanism of cellular injury from the following causes: hypoxia, free radicals and reactive oxygen species, infectious agents, inflammatory and immune responses, genetic factors, insufficient nutrients, and physical trauma.

4. Identify cellular accumulations that may occur as manifestations of cellular injury.

5. Compare dystrophic and metastatic calcification.

6. Discuss apoptosis.

7. Describe normal, endogenous pigments.

8. Describe the four major types of necrosis and give examples of the tissue types affected by each.

9. Discuss the cellular mechanisms of normal aging.

10. Identify the clinical manifestations of somatic death.

LECTURE OUTLINE	INSTRUCTOR'S NOTES

Cellular Adaptation
  Atrophy
  Hypertrophy
  Hyperplasia
  Dysplasia
  Metaplasia
Cellular Injury
  General mechanisms of cell injury
  Hypoxic injury
  Free radicals and reactive oxygen species injury
  Mechanisms of chemical injury
  Unintentional and intentional injuries
  Infectious injury
  Immunologic and inflammatory injury
Manifestations of Cellular Injury
  Water
  Lipids and carbohydrates
  Glycogen
  Proteins

LECTURE OUTLINE	INSTRUCTOR'S NOTES

Pigments
    Calcium
    Urate
    Systemic manifestations
Cellular Death
    Necrosis
    Apoptosis
Aging and altered cellular and tissue biology
    Normal life span
    Life expectancy and gender differences
    Theories and mechanisms of aging
    Cellular aging
    Tissue and systemic aging
Somatic Death

DIFFICULT CONCEPTS

Cellular Adaptation

Like people, cells adapt to their environment. Adaptation is protection. When a cell is threatened, for example, it is no longer receiving food or nourishment, and it starts to "digest parts of itself" or becomes atrophic. This process involves proliferation of autophagic vacuoles that ultimately leads to lysosomal damage and a decrease in cellular size. This response is protective because the injured organelles are essentially sacrificed so that the uninjured organelles can continue to thrive. The adaptive processes of atrophy, hypertrophy, hyperplasia, and metaplasia can all be discussed in the context of protection and "social control." Individual cells are members of a complex cellular society where survival of the entire organism, not survival or proliferation of the individual cell, is key. When severe or long-term stressors (prolonged starvation) overwhelm adaptive processes, cellular injury or death ensues.

Cellular Injury as a Process

It is often difficult for students to view cellular injury as an ongoing, continuous process rather than a single, isolated event. Discussing the process of hypoxic injury helps students discern the "specific events" as well as the "bridges" or "connections" of the different events into an ongoing continuum. For example, a decrease in oxygen leads to a decrease in oxidative phosphorylation (ATP), which leads to the dissolution of intracellular membranes because of the movement of water into the cell. The movement of water into the cell occurs because the decrease in ATP causes the failure of ATP pumping, resulting in an increased intracellular Na^+ and Ca^{++}; water can then freely enter the cell. Dissolution of all cellular membranes is occurring simultaneously.

Free Radicals

The concept of damaging free radicals has been exploited by the mass media. Much of the students knowledge of free radicals may have come from the media. Students need to know that current research is still incomplete and a complete understanding is lacking. When presenting the concepts, be sure the students know that media-hyped quick fixes (like megadose vitamins) are unproven and controversial.

CRITICAL THINKING

1. Ms. Jones has an annual pap smear and gynecologic exam. Three years ago, immediately prior to her third pregnancy, the pathology report of her pap smear indicated she had hormonal hyperplasia. Her current pap smear indicates she has atypical hyperplasia or dysplasia. What is the difference between these?

   Answer: Hyperplasia is an increase in the number of normal cells. In this situation, Ms. Jones had normal hormonal hyperplasia due to increased cellular division. Estrogen was stimulating the uterine endometrium to grow and thicken in preparation for the ovum's implantation. Dysplasia or atypical hyperplasia is an abnormal change in the size, shape, or organization of mature cells. It most commonly occurs in epithelial membranes such as the uterus. It is strongly associated with neoplasia (malignant growth). Most frequently women with uterine dysplasia will have further testing done, which may include a biopsy.

2. Ms. Rawlins is a 28 year old alcoholic. She is admitted in labor and delivers a baby girl. The child is placed in foster care. What signs and symptoms would you look for of fetal alcohol syndrome during the first year of the child's life?

   Answer: Congenital abnormalities seen in children with fetal alcohol syndrome include: microcephaly, low birth weight, cardiovascular defects, developmental disabilities, mental retardation, thinned upper lip, small eye openings (palpebral fissues), epicanthal folds, and receded upper jaw (retrognathia).

Fluids and Electrolytes, Acids and Bases

OBJECTIVES

After review of this chapter, the learner will be able to:

1. Discuss the two functional fluid compartments of the body.

2. Describe the causation, pathophysiologic process, and clinical manifestations of edema.

3. Discuss the regulatory processes for sodium and water balance in the body, including the role of antidiuretic hormone, aldosterone, renin, angiotensin, and atrial natriuretic hormone.

4. Define hypotonic, isotonic, and hypertonic alterations in water balance and give an example of each.

5. Identify the basic causes of hyper- and hyponatremia and chloremia.

6. Discuss potassium with regard to function, distribution, regulation, and pathophysiologic imbalances.

7. Discuss the role of hydrogen ion concentration in cellular function and dysfunction.

8. Explain how the lungs and the kidneys regulate acid-base balance.

9. Differentiate between respiratory and metabolic acid-base disorders.

LECTURE OUTLINE	INSTRUCTOR'S NOTES

Distribution of Body Fluids
    Maturation and the Distribution of Body Fluids
    Water Movement Between ICF and ECF
    Water Movement Between Plasma and Interstitial
        Fluid
Alterations in Water Movement
    Edema
Sodium, Chloride, and Water Balance
    Water balance
    Sodium and chloride balance
Alterations in Sodium, Chloride, and Water Balance
    Isotonic alterations (fluid volume deficits)
    Hypertonic alterations
        Hypernatremia
        Water deficit
        Hyperchloremia
    Hypotonic alterations
        Hyponatremia
        Water excess
        Hypochloremia

LECTURE OUTLINE	INSTRUCTOR'S NOTES

Alterations in Potassium and Other Electrolytes
    Potassium
        Hypokalemia
        Hyperkalemia
Other Electrolytes
Acid-Base Balance
    Hydrogen ion and pH
    Buffer systems
        Carbonic acid-bicarbonate buffering
        Protein buffering
        Renal buffering
    Acid-base imbalances
        Metabolic acidosis
        Metabolic alkalosis
        Respiratory acidosis
        Respiratory alkalosis

DIFFICULT CONCEPTS

Regulation of Water Movement Across Membranes

Helping students understand that osmotic and oncotic pressures are pulling pressures in relation to water and that hydrostatic pressure is a pushing pressure in relation to water helps them to understand how water moves in relation to these different forces. Once students understand the rationale behind forces of hydrostatic pressure and osmotic pressure, they then have a basis for predicting fluid movement under both normal and abnormal conditions.

Differentiating Between Compensation and Correction of Acid-Base Disturbances

The buffer systems of the body have the same general function of acting to stabilize pH. The plasma buffer systems act in seconds, whereas the respiratory system responds in minutes. The renal system is more powerful but acts over a period of hours to days. Each system has a differing capacity to compensate or correct for respiratory or metabolic acid-base disorders. Respiratory compensation for a primary metabolic acid-base disorder can be initiated quickly, much like a small aircraft which can rapidly be put into service but can carry a limited number of passengers. The respiratory system can compensate for a metabolic disorder but requires the kidneys to fully correct it. Chronic respiratory acid-base disturbances can be fully compensated by renal activity, but the ultimate correction must occur through the regulation of carbon dioxide, which is achieved in the lungs. The kidneys, in this case, can be thought of as jumbo jets which can carry large volumes over long distances.

As a general rule, primary respiratory acid-base disorders are compensated by renal function, and primary metabolic acid-base disorders are compensated by the lungs. Correction of primary respiratory acid-base disorders requires adequate respiratory function, and correction of primary metabolic acid-base disorders requires adequate renal function.

CRITICAL THINKING

1. Ms. Brown is an elderly female diabetic who was too ill to get out of bed for two days. She has had a severe cough and has been unable to eat or drink during this time. On admission her laboratory values show:

   Sodium (Na^+) 156
   Potassium (K^+) 4
   Chloride (Cl^-) 115
   Arterial blood gases: pH 7.30; pCO_2 40; pO_2 70; HCO_3^- 20

   a. What type of water and solute imbalance does Ms. Brown have?

   b. What symptoms would you expect to find?

   c. What would be the treatment?

   d. What do her ABGs mean?

   e. Does she have an anion gap?

Answers:

a. Ms. Brown has a hypertonic imbalance with a high solute extracellular fluid (ECF) concentration. This means that ECF water has been lost and there is shifting of water from the intracellular space into the extracellular space. Ms. Brown's solute imbalance is hypernatremic, because her sodium level is greater than 147 mEq/L. Her hypernatremia is caused by water losses due to a combination of her pulmonary illness and diabetes mellitus.

b. Her symptoms would include thirst, fever, dry mucous membranes, restlessness, tachycardia, postural hypotension, weight loss, weak pulses, decreased urine output, convulsions, and possible cerebral hemorrhage.

c. Treatment of hypernatremia includes giving a salt-free, isotonic fluid such as D5W until the serum sodium level returns to normal.

d. Ms. Brown also has a metabolic acidosis, because her pH is below 7.35, her pCO_2 is normal, and her HCO_3^- is less than 24 mEq/L. She is also hypoxic, indicated by a pO_2 of less than 80.

e. To calculate her anion gap: $[Na^+(156) + K^+(4)] - [HCO_3^-(20) + Cl^-(115)] = 25$ mEq/L. Normal anion gap is 10-12 mEq/L. Therefore, Ms. Brown has a positive anion gap. This means she has an acidosis associated with anion other than chloride. In her situation, she has acidosis as a result of her ketosis and/or starvation. Treatment of her metabolic acidosis and hypoxia would include giving her oxygen, checking her blood glucose level, and possibly giving her insulin. She will also need nutritional supplementation.

2. Mr. Appel has severe chronic obstructive pulmonary disease (COPD). He is admitted to the hospital with the complaint of increasing dyspnea, increased sputum, anxiety, and diaphoresis. He states he feels weak and tired. He routinely takes a diuretic (furosemide) and his pulmonary medications. The following laboratory values are obtained:

   Arterial blood gases: pH 7.25; pO_2 60; pCO_2 78; HCO_3^- 30
   Sodium (Na^+) 140 mEq/L
   Potassium (K^+) 2.0 mEq/L
   Chloride (Cl^-) 105 mEq/L

   a. What type of imbalance does Mr. Brown have?

   b. Interpret his ABGs.

   c. What would be the treatment?

Answers:

a. Mr. Appel has hypokalemia, indicated by a potassium (K^+) level of less than 3.5 mEq/L.

b. He also has respiratory acidosis, because his pH is less than 7.35 and his pCO_2 is greater than 45. His HCO_3^- is elevated in an attempt to compensate for the high pCO_2, but it is not enough to keep his pH within normal limits. He is also hypoxic because his pO_2 is less than 80. His sodium and chloride are within normal limits.

c. Mr. Brown would need supplemental oxygen, oral or IV replacement of potassium (i.e., K-dur po or D5.2NS with 20 mEq/L), restoration of adequate alveolar ventilation to remove excess CO_2 via nebulizer treatments or metered dose inhalers, and treatment of any pulmonary infection. If his pulmonary status does not improve, mechanical ventilation may be necessary.

CHAPTER

5

Immunity

OBJECTIVES

After review of this chapter, the learner will be able to:

1. Define primary and secondary immune response.

2. Define antigen and describe between the various types of antigens.

3. Define and describe humoral and cell-mediated immunity.

4. Describe the antibodies with a focus on origin, functions, and specificity.

5. Discuss the significance of HLA in defending the body.

6. Explain the clonal selection theory.

7. Diagram the development of five types of T-cells from stem cells.

8. Describe the immune response.

9. Discuss in general the overall function of cytokines.

10. Describe the steps of antigen processing.

11. Discuss the alterations in immunity for infants and the elderly.

LECTURE OUTLINE	INSTRUCTOR'S NOTES

Characteristics of the Immune Response
    Natural versus acquired immunity
    Primary and secondary immune responses
    Humoral versus cell-mediated immunity
Induction of the Immune Response
    Antigens
    Histocompatibility antigens
        HLA complex
        Role of HLA antigens
    Blood group antigens
        Rh system
        ABO system
Humoral Immune Response
    B lymphocytes
    Immunoglobulins
        Structure of immunoglobulin molecules
        Function of antibodies
        Classes of immunoglobulins
        Monoclonal antibodies
    Secretory immune system
Cell-Mediated Immune Response

LECTURE OUTLINE	INSTRUCTOR'S NOTES

Cellular Interactions in the Immune Response
   Cytokines
   Antigen processing, presentation, and recognition
   T-cell and B-cell differentiation
      T-cell differentiation
      B-cell differentiation
   Control of B- and T-cell development
Pediatric Immune Function
Aging Immune Function

DIFFICULT CONCEPTS

Histocompatibility

For this concept, use the analogy of an ID bracelet. Just like an ID bracelet, cells carry identification or "codes" that help distinguish each individual's tissue from the tissue of others. Explain that the code corresponds to the major histocompatibility antigens (HLA antigens). Specifically, however, point out that just like several different kinds of ID bracelets (some with initials or names and some for red alert or identifying a person as a diabetic), not all cells use the same code. For example, red blood cells do not have the A, B, C allele but use the ABO and Rh factor antigens. This analogy is helpful in explaining the structure and function of the HLA antigens.

Antigen Processing and the Role of Cytokines

Cellular interactions in the immune response is a topic that usually requires repetitive explanations. Again, the analogy of the cell as a "social organism" is helpful. Use concepts such as affability, operator assistance, conversation, messengers, control center, and so on. Begin this discussion slowly by defining all the "talkers," antigens, immunogens, antigen-presenting cells, cytokines, HLA class I and II antigens, CD3 complex, and T-cell receptor. Draw the entire "conversation" on the board using transparencies for specifics. Students usually "get it" through constant reinforcement of the importance of conversation. For example, the particular HLA class that bears the antigen helps determine which cell will "respond" to the presentation of the antigen.

CRITICAL THINKING

1. Mr. Jones becomes infected with the HIV virus on Friday night. The following Monday he donates a unit of blood. The HIV test is an antibody test. Will his blood test positive for the virus? Why?

   Answer: No, there is a lag time between antigen introduction and antibody production.

Inflammation

OBJECTIVES

After review of this chapter, the learner will be able to:

1. Define inflammation and state the major limitation of the response.

2. Discuss the microscopic findings in inflammation and relate those to the macroscopic manifestations of an inflammatory response.

3. Describe the role of the mast cell in the activation of inflammation, including the effects of histamine and serotonin.

4. Identify the three plasma protein systems which mediate the inflammation response.

5. Diagram the complement system cascade, including activation via both the classical and alternative pathways.

6. Discuss each of the cell types involved in the inflammation response by role and relative importance to the process.

7. Describe the interruptions in the inflammatory process occurring with deficiencies of each of the cell types discussed above.

8. Compare and contrast the origin and roles of cytokines, particularly lymphokines, interferons, and interleukins, in the inflammation response.

9. Differentiate between local and systemic inflammation responses on the basis of clinical manifestations.

10. Describe healing by primary and secondary intention.

LECTURE OUTLINE	INSTRUCTOR'S NOTES

The Acute Inflammatory Response
The Mast Cell
    Degranulation of vasoactive amines and chemotactic factors
    Synthesis of leukotrienes and prostaglandins
Plasma Protein Systems
    The complement system
        Classic pathway
        Alternative pathway
    Clotting system
    Kinin system
    Control and interaction of plasma protein systems

LECTURE OUTLINE	INSTRUCTOR'S NOTES

Cellular Components of Inflammation
    Function of phagocytes
    Polymorphonuclear neutrophils
    Monocytes and macrophages
    Eosinophils
Cellular Products
    Infammatory cytokines
    Interferons
Systemic Manifestations of Acute Inflammation
Chronic Inflammation
Local Manifestations of Inflammation
Resolution and Repair
    Reconstructive phase
    Maturation phase
Dysfunctional Wound Healing
    Dysfunction during the inflammatory response
    Dysfunction during the reconstructive phase

DIFFICULT CONCEPTS

The Complexity of the Inflammatory Response

    The inflammatory response is complex because of the different cells, inflammatory mediators, and protein systems that are involved. Students are motivated to learn about inflammation when they understand how generalizable the process is to any type of injury or disease and its essential role in regeneration and repair of tissue. Figure 6-3 is a helpful summary of inflammation and represents the interaction between cells of inflammation and the vascular response. This content is taught early in the term and begins with the cells and their function in sequence (mast cells, platelets, neutrophils, macrophages, and fibroblasts) combined with what is happening with the changes in the vasculature. This helps with understanding the local and protective symptoms of inflammation (redness, heat, pain, edema/swelling, and loss of function). The protein systems (clotting, complements, and kinins) and their role in sustaining and controlling inflammation are introduced next. The stage is then set to present the phases of wound healing with generalization of the whole process of inflammation to different types of wounds: for example, lacerations, myocardial infarction, glomerulonephritis, or pneumonia. Students particularly enjoy working in small groups with large sheets of paper to make concept maps linking the components of inflammation to a specific type of injury. The major concepts are then reviewed when students are learning about specific pathophysiologies later in the term.

CRITICAL THINKING

1. Your patient is having an acute inflammatory response. List 3 tests that can be used to confirm this.

    Answer:
    1. Temperature measurement--Acute inflammation produces fever.
    2. Leucocyte count--Leucocytes, particularly neutrophils, increase in acute inflammation. This results in a higher-than-normal percentage of immature neutrophils.
    3. Erythrocyte sedimentation rate--It is increased during acute inflamation.

Hypersensitivities, Infection, and Immunodeficiencies

OBJECTIVES

After review of this chapter, the learner will be able to:

1. Define the three stimuli of hypersensitivity: autoimmunity, isoimmunity, and allergy.

2. Compare the four mechanisms of hypersensitivity.

3. Differentiate between immediate and delayed hypersensitivities and give an example of each.

4. Define autoimmune diseases and give examples.

5. Describe the four types of hypersensitivity reactions.

6. Compare autoimmunity with alloimmunity.

7. Describe the factors influencing infection by a pathogen.

8. Compare bacterial, viral, and fungal infections.

9. Describe countermeasures against pathogens.

10. Describe congenital and acquired immune deficiencies.

11. Discuss the pathogenesis of acquired immune deficiency syndrome (AIDS).

12. Describe the treatment for AIDS.

LECTURE OUTLINE	INSTRUCTOR'S NOTES

Alterations in Immunity and Inflammation
    Hypersensitivity: allergy, autoimmunity, and
        alloimmunity
        Mechanisms of hypersensitivity
            IgE-mediated reactions
            Tissue-specific reactions
            Immune-complex-mediated injury
            Cell-mediated tissue destruction
        Targets of hypersensitivity
            Allergy
            Autoimmunity
            Alloimmunity
        Autoimmune and alloimmune diseases
            Systemic lupus erythematosus
            Graft rejection
Infection
    Microorganisms and humans: a dynamic
        relationship
    Classes of infectious organisms

LECTURE OUTLINE	INSTRUCTOR'S NOTES

Innate host resistance mechanisms
Pathogenic defense mechanisms
Infection and injury
    Bacterial
    Viral
    Fungal
Clinical manifestations
Countermeasures against pathogen defenses
Recent pathogenic adaptations
The future
Immunodeficiencies
    Congenital immunodeficiencies
    Acquired immunodeficiencies
        Nutritional deficiencies
        Iatrogenic deficiencies
        Deficiencies caused by trauma
        Deficiencies caused by stress
        Acquired immune deficiency syndrome (AIDS)
    Clinical evaluation of immunity
    Replacement therapies for immune deficiencies

DIFFICULT CONCEPTS

Hypersensitivity Reactions and Cell Interactions

What is difficult in understanding each of the hypersensitivity reactions are the interactions, or "communications," among the immune cells. For example, in type II hypersensitivity, it is the interaction among antibody, tissue-specific antigens, and complement-mediated lysis. How all of these cells "interact"—and what activates what—are difficult concepts. In addition, understanding the anatomy and function of antibody—where on the antibody complement attaches or "fixes"—is prerequisite to understanding the entire lytic mechanism. Mastery of several prerequisite concepts is necessary: the role of macrophages, the role of neutrophils, T-lymphocytes and B-lymphocytes, and so on. (Normal immunity is included as a major topic in pathophysiology courses.)

Autoimmunity

Because the exact mechanisms of the autoimmune response is unknown, this concept may present difficulty. The interaction of genetic predisposition and environmental factors has been documented in some autoimmune diseases. This association in other diseases is less clear. What is known is that autoimmune diseases are familial. Genetic research may eventually yield the key to further understanding.

CRITICAL THINKING

1. Diagram what happens during a type I hypersensitivity reaction and indicate responses to major mediators.

   Answer:

   Exposure to Allergen

   Cross-linking of adjacent IgE receptors on mast cells

   Release of preformed and newly formed mediators:

   Excess IgE:
   binds to receptors on circulating basophils, mast cells, and other effector cells, causing further degranulation

   Histamine:
   H1 receptor: increased vascular permeability, vasodilation, urticaria formation, bronchial constriction with wheezing and coughing, increased gut permeability

   H2 receptor: decreasing degranulation, increasing lymphocyte activation, decreased neutrophil chemotaxis and enzyme release

   Proteolytic enzymes, kininogenase and tryptase:
   activate the kinin pathway and C3, which trigger the complement cascade

   Heparin:
   decreases clot formation

   Chemotactic factors:
   call or activate other inflammatory and immune cells, such as eosinophil chemotactic factor of anaphylaxis ECF-A, platelet activating factor (PAF)

   SRS-A (Slow reacting substance of anaphylaxis):
   smooth muscle contraction and increased vascular permeability

   Clinical Manifestations

   GI: vomiting, diarrhea, abdominal pain, malabsorption
   Skin: urticaria, itching, angioedema
   Respiratory: conjunctivitis, rhinitis, bronchospasm, asthma, laryngeal edema
   CV: hypotension, tachycardia, dysrhythmias

2. Analyze the difference between the antigen-antibody reaction in a type II hypersensitivity reaction and a type III hypersensitivity reaction. Give an example of each type of reaction.

Answer: Type II hypersensitivity reaction is also known as cytotoxic or cytolytic hypersensitivity reaction. It is characterized by antibodies that attack antigens on the surface of specific cells or tissues. The reaction is organ specific. This antigen-antibody reaction is immediate, occurring within fifteen to thirty minutes after exposure to the antigen. IgG and IgM are the principal antibodies. It is mediated by the complement system and a variety of principal effector cells including tissue macrophages, platelets, killer cells, neutrophils, and eosinophils. The symptoms are related to the antigenic target of the antibody. Examples of this type of hypersensitivity reaction include ABO transfusion reactions, hemolytic disease of the newborn, myasthenia gravis, thyroiditis, hyperacute graft rejections, and autoimmune hemolytic anemias.

Type III hypersensitivity reaction is also known as immune complex or arthus disease. This reaction is a sequential process beginning with an interaction between a soluble antigen and soluble antibody. It is characterized by antigen-antibody complex formation that usually occurs in the circulation. The complex is then deposited into vascular walls or extravascular tissues, causing an inflammatory reaction. The reaction is not organ specific and peaks six hours after exposure to the antigen. IgG is the principal antibody. The principal effector cells include neutrophils and mast cells. Examples of this type of hypersensitivity reaction include serum sickness, gomerulonephritis, systemic lupus erythematosus, rheumatoid arthritis, drug-induced vasculitis, serum sickness, and polyarteritis nodosa.

3. Explain why people with acquired immune deficiency syndrome (AIDS) develop opportunistic infections.

Answer: People with AIDS are infected with the human immunodeficiency virus. This RNA virus is attracted to cells with CD4 receptors on their surface. The CD4 receptor is found on T-cells, microglial cells, lymph nodes, alveolar macrophages, thymus gland, bone marrow, and Langerhans cells in the skin. Other cells also infected by HIV include glial cells in the brain, endothelial cells, cervical cells, retinal cells, transformed B-cells, and bone marrow-derived circulating dendritic cells and enterochromaffin cells in the colon, duodenum, and rectum. As a result, people with AIDS are deficient in CD4 cells—especially T-cells. Without T-helper cells (CD4), the immune system is not effective. T-helper cells secrete lymphokines that call B-cells and other inflammatory cells to the sites of infection and stimulate functioning B-cells to manufacture antibodies. Therefore, people with AIDS are lacking the cells necessary to recognize and fight infection.

Stress and Disease

OBJECTIVES

After review of this chapter, the learner will be able to:

1. Describe the physiologic basis of the general adaptation syndrome (GAS) as proposed by Selye.

2. Discuss the components of physiologic stress and the stages of the GAS response.

3. Define dynamic steady state and discuss the role of a physiologic response to stress in its maintenance.

4. Discuss the neuroendocrine response to stress from initiation by recognition of a stressor through resolution by exhaustion or adaptation.

5. List the effects of cortisol, epinephrine, and norepinephrine on the individual under stress.

6. Describe the known mechanisms of interaction between the neuroendocrine and immune responses to stress.

7. Identify other hormones affected by the physiologic response to a stressor.

8. Apply understanding of the stress response to a clinical or personal situation by description of the factors involved in the initiation of the response and manifestations observed or experienced.

9. Discuss the factors which mediate an individual's ability to cope with a stressor.

LECTURE OUTLINE

INSTRUCTOR'S NOTES

Concepts of Stress
    General adaptation syndrome
    Psychologic mediators and specificity
    Homeostasis as a dynamic steady state
Thc Stress Response
    Psychoneuroimmunologic regulation
    Neuroendocrine regulation
        Catecholamines
        Cortisol
        Other hormones
    Role of the immune system
Stress, Coping, and Illness

DIFFICULT CONCEPTS

Concept of Stress

The concept of stress as interactional or transactional helps students understand that situations, per se, are not necessarily stressful, but how people appraise and react to them are stressful. It is difficult but important to help students move beyond the classic stress triad (general adaptation syndrome) to the interactions involved in the entire psychoneuroimmunologic response.

Regulatory Interactions of the Stress Response

Most students have heard of the interaction of the autonomic nervous system, the pituitary gland, and the adrenal gland in the stress response. New for most of them are the links with the immune system. Again, the concepts of communication and pathways that appear to regulate "communication" between these systems with both direct and indirect patterned effects should be stressed. However, the specific stress-induced mechanisms causing different kinds of illnesses are not clearly defined. Many students are surprised to learn how various hormones, neurotransmitters, and neuropeptides potentially affect immune cells and, conversely, how immune cell-derived cytokines and other products affect neurocrine and endocrine cells.

CRITICAL THINKING

1. Explain what physiologic actions catecholamines and cortisol have in common and in what ways they differ in their actions.

   Answer: Cortisol and the catecholamines affect the cardiovascular system by increasing cardiac output and increasing blood pressure. They increase lipolysis and gluconeogenesis in the liver, leading to increased blood glucose and free fatty acids. Increased blood glucose by catecholamines requires cortisol (glucocorticoids) for maximal activity. They also increase protein breakdown in lymphoid tissue, causing lymphoid tissue atrophy.

   In contrast to cortisol, catecholamines also affect the pulmonary system by dilating bronchial airways, increasing ventilation, and increasing oxygen supply. They affect the GI system by decreasing gastric secretion. Pancreatic effects include decreased insulin and increased glucagon, leading to increased blood glucose. They decrease blood to the skin while increasing blood flow to the brain. Catecholamines also increase glycogenolysis and contraction in muscle tissue.

   Cortisol acts to increase protein catabolism and blood levels of amino acids in most body tissues except in the liver, where it increases the rate of synthesis of proteins and RNA. It affects the immune system by increasing circulating polymorphonuclear leukocytes (PMNs) and by decreasing all other white blood cells, immunoglobulin production, and release of kinins, prostaglandins, and histamines.

2. You are caring for a 29-year-old female who is married with two small children, ages 1 and 3, at home. She is recuperating from a left lower lobectomy for bronchogenic carcinoma. Although her chest x-rays show full lung expansion, she has a persistent air leak. Therefore, she continues to need a chest tube to suction and must remain hospitalized. Six days post-op, she is sad, depressed, and not eating. She states that she does not feel she will ever get better or go home. How would you use your knowledge of the coping process to help her?

   Answer: You need to explain that her emotions act as a stressor which causes her immune and endocrine systems to increase the likelihood of continuing illness. Stressor models indicate that ineffective coping can lead to illness. You must teach and encourage her to use therapeutic relaxation and visualization to decrease stress and increase coping.

CHAPTER

9

Biology of Cancer

OBJECTIVES

After review of this chapter, the learner will be able to:

1. Identify the two mutational routes resulting in uncontrolled cellular proliferation.

2. Cancer is defined by two heritable properties, autonomy and anaplasia. Describe these properties.

3. Discuss in general cell surface changes and their functional importance in cancer.

4. Define proto-oncogene, cellular oncogene (c^+ onc), viral oncogene (v- onc), and tumor suppressor gene.

5. Discuss the initiation-promotion-progression model of carcinogenesis.

6. Summarize the effects of ionizing radiation on carcinogenesis.

7. Discuss the relationship between hormones and human cancer.

8. Describe in general the tumor immune surveillance theory.

9. Discuss immunologic defense against tumors.

10. Describe ways that tumors escape immunologic rejection.

LECTURE OUTLINE	INSTRUCTOR'S NOTES

Cancer: A Disease of Growth, Division, and Cell
    Differentiation
    Social control genes and cellular division
    Cell differentiation
    Tumor classification and nomenclature
Characteristics of Cancer Cells
    Cell surface changes and their functional
        importance
        Glycolipids and glycoproteins
        Altered membrane transport of permeability
        Protease
        Altered anchoring junctions and gap junctions
    Tumor cell markers
    Intercellular changes in cancer cells
        Cytoskeleton
        Cytoplasmic organelles and altered metabolism
        Density-dependent inhibition of growth
        Growth requirements: inducers of differentia-
            tion

| **LECTURE OUTLINE** | **INSTRUCTOR'S NOTES** |

Autocrine stimulation hypothesis
Changes in the nucleus and cell protein
The Causes of Cancer
Genetics and cancer families
Gene-environment interaction
Oncogenic viruses
Tumor suppressor genes
Carcinogenesis
Monoclonal origin
Cell accidents: a requisite for cancer development
The slow stages of cancer development
Oncogenes and tumor-suppressor genes
Stem cell or blocked differentiation
Intercellular communication
Initiation-promotion-progression theory of
carcinogenesis
Environmental risk factors
Hormones
Immunobiology of Cancer
Tumor immune surveillance theory
Tumor antigens
Immunologic defense against tumors

DIFFICULT CONCEPTS

Social Control Genes and Uncontrolled Cell Proliferation

Once again, using the analogy of a cellular society, it is relevant to point out that the overall goal of this society is survival of the entire organism and not just the individual cell. Therefore, a balance is maintained between cell birth rate and cell death rate. The cellular control mechanisms that regulate cell birth and cell death are called "social controls" and require "social control genes." These genes (oncogenes and tumor-suppressor genes) control growth-factor-regulated cell division. Mutation of these genes causes tumor formation.

Anchorage Independence

This is usually a new concept for students. Anchoring junctions connect the cytoskeleton, the "bones and muscles" of the cell, to its neighbor cell or the extracellular matrix. Cancer cells exhibit anchorage-independence with decreased cell-cell and cell-extracellular attachments. The cell is allowed to metastasize without anchorage. Unlike normal cells, tumor cells continue to divide when they are missing the necessary components for anchorage.

Tumor Immune Surveillance Theory

The entire area of immunity and cancer is a difficult concept. It is very difficult if students have not had a strong, recent review of normal immunity and, thus, are confused even by terminology. Introduce (with examples) the idea that immune-suppressed individuals have an increased risk of developing certain types of tumors. Then ask students what the requirements are for the body to mount a successful immune response; they usually respond with the notion of antigen or something that is identified by lymphocytes as foreign. A discussion follows on tumor antigens, identification of tumor-reactive antibodies in the serum of some individuals with cancer, immunologic defense against tumors, and the theorized tumor immune surveillance escape mechanisms.

CRITICAL THINKING

1. Ms. Johans has a Grade I tumor of the lung. Mr. Tompkins has a Grade IV tumor of the lung. Explain how these tumors are similar and how they differ.

   Answer: Both tumors show a local increase in atypical cells that grow rapidly. They have lost their normal cellular arrangement and differentiation. Their cellular components and structure differ from that of the tissue of origin; they have increased nuclear size, increased mitoses, and variable cell shape and size. Cancer cells also lose density-dependent inhibition of growth, so they pile up and form irregular masses. Vascularity is increased to aid tumor growth. Both tumors might be expected to produce an ectopic hormone such as adrenocorticotropic hormone or antidiuretic hormone.

   The difference between the tumors is reflected in their grading. A Grade I tumor is well differentiated and closely resembles the tissue of origin. A Grade IV tumor has no resemblance to the tissue of origin and is very poorly differentiated.

2. Mr. Benson, 60 years old, lives near phosphate and uranium deposits. His father was a uranium miner. Mr. Benson has worked in a phosphate processing plant since his early twenties. (Phosphate ore is combined with low grade uranium and emits constant low alpha radiation.) He is a pack-a-day smoker and drinks alcohol moderately. He describes himself as a "meat and potatoes man" and likes to barbecue. Using the initiation-promotion-progression theory, explain his lung tumor development and analyze factors that contributed to each stage.

   Answer: According to this theory, cancer involves multiple stages including initiation, promotion, and progression. This theory best explains cancers in adults with a 20+ year latency period. In the initiation stage, there is rapid, irreversible altering or mutation of DNA that occurs after a single exposure to a carcinogen (initiator). There must be a strong enough dose or exposure to cause DNA change. In this case, Mr. Benson was most likely exposed to ionizing radiation as a child—perhaps inadvertent exposure due to his father's occupation.

   After this initiation stage, the cells stay dormant in G_0 phase or, if dividing, produce very small numbers of transformed daughter cells. The initiated cells are not considered cancerous until a promoting agent acts on them over time to produce an altered, autonomous phenotype.

   In the promotion stage, promoters induce tumor development. These promoters can be hormones, chemical agents such as drugs, chemicals, tobacco, and plant products, or environmental factors such as air pollution, occupation, diet, and UV radiation. In order for promoters to induce tumor development, there must be time-dependent repeated exposures to the promoters or prolonged exposure over a period of time. Promoters interfere with differentiation and maturation, activating the transformed cell to go through mitotic division and continue to go through replication phases. In the early stages, the effects of promoters can be reversible.

   In Mr. Benson's case, he had a number of possible promoters that contributed to his cancer, including smoking, alcohol use, occupational exposure to fine dust particles, chronic exposure to alpha radiation, a high meat and fat diet, and polycyclic hydrocarbons produced from meat charred as a result of barbecue use.

   In the progression stage, there are chromosomal abnormalities in the cells. The greater the replications, the more the cell becomes abnormal. This leads to tumor development, invasion, and metastasis.

3. Present an argument for why one 60-year-old individual develops cancer and another 60-year-old with identical promoters does not develop cancer.

Answer: Tumor cells are parasites that are capable of bypassing the host's immune surveillance potential. Even with the same promoters, individuals with normal immunocompetence can develop tumors. There are several hypothesized escape mechanisms including antigenic modulation, tumor secretion of immunosuppressive substances, escape, blocking antibodies or factors, immunostimulation, and T-suppressor cells.

Antigenic modulation occurs when tumor cells down-regulate their expression of cell surface molecules when grown in the presence of certain antibodies. Tumors can secrete immunosuppressive substances that block necessary cellular immune interactions. They can either directly inhibit lymphocyte activation or interfere with other immune functions.

Tumor cells can escape or sneak through immunologic detection. Escape can occur when daughter cells lose or modify tumor antigen in a heterogenous mixture of cells. Tumor cells can sneak through when there is a small amount of tumor-associated antigen. This small amount of antigen is too small to elicit an immune response. The cells continue to grow until the tumor mass is too large with too many rapidly growing cells to be eliminated by the immune system.

Tumors can secrete blocking antibodies or factors. These antibodies are TAA specific but are incapable of functioning in an ADCC response or lysing tumor by fixing complement. In either case, the antibody/antigen formation cannot be processed by the appropriate antigen-presenting cells.

There is an optimal tumor: cytotoxic, or killer (Tc), cell ratio or balance. Small numbers of Tc cells increase cancer cell growth while large numbers of Tc cells decrease tumor growth.

Tumors can cause the induction of T-suppressor (Ts) cells which are antigen-specific. These cells turn off the immune system, block other types of immune responses, or mediate a modification in the magnitude or type of immune response elicited. This strategy works because the immune system is unable to determine whether the actively dividing cell is detrimental (e.g., tumor) or beneficial (e.g., bone marrow) to the host. Activated macrophages have also been reported to exert suppressive activity that is nonspecific in origin.

Tumor Spread

OBJECTIVES

After review of this chapter, the learner will be able to:

1. Describe the mechanisms of tumor invasion.

2. Discuss the three-step theory of invasion.

3. Discuss the factors implicated in metastasis of tumors: rate of growth, angiogenesis, lack of cellular adhesion, and absence of cellular barriers.

4. Describe the clinical manifestations of cancer.

5. Describe the treatment strategies for cancer.

LECTURE OUTLINE	INSTRUCTOR'S NOTES

Tumor Spread
    Local spread
        Cellular multiplication
        Mechanical invasion
        Lytic enzymes
        Decreased cell adhesion
        Increased motility
    The three-step theory of invasion
    Patterns of spread: metastasis
        Direct or continuous extension
        Metastasis by lymphatics and bloodstream
        Angiogenesis and angiogenesis factors
        Growth of metastases and metastatic potential
        Distribution and common sites of distant metastases
        Staging
Clinical Manifestations of Cancer
    Pain
    Fatigue
    Cachexia
    Anemia
    Leukopenia and thrombocytopenia
    Infection
Cancer Treatment
    Chemotherapy
    Radiation
    Surgery
    Immunotherapy

DIFFICULT CONCEPTS

Three-Step Theory of Invasion

If students understand the characteristics of a cancer cell (e.g., anchorage-independence, lytic enzymes, etc.), this section is not difficult; it just contains new information. Figure 10-2 is helpful in illustrating the three steps: attachment through laminin and anchorage to the laminin receptor; secretion of proteolytic enzymes, specifically type IV collagenase; and tumor cell locomotion. Figure 10-3 is a slide of an actual breast cancer cell showing pseudopodia, the fingerlike projections that facilitate movement.

Immunotherapy

Immunotherapy is difficult because it requires mastery of many concepts in normal immunity. Stressing the three mechanisms that describe the activities of the biological response modifiers using illustrations from the text is helpful. The three mechanisms are (1) direct cytotoxic effects on cancer cells (e.g., interferon), (2) initiation or augmentation of the host's tumor-immune rejection response (Figure 10-5), and (3) modification of cancer cell susceptibility to the lytic or tumor-static effects of the immune system (Figure 10-6).

CRITICAL THINKING

1. If Ms. Fuentes has breast cancer, how would angiogenesis and invasion influence tumor growth and metastasis?

   Answer: Angiogenesis influences cancer growth by increasing tumor vascularity. Increased vascularity brings nutrients and oxygen needed for cell growth directly to the tumor. This causes a spurt in tumor growth because the cells do not have to wait for nutrients to diffuse via the interstitial space. Tumor cells may secrete growth factors, prostaglandin E1, proteolytic enzymes, and possibly tumor angiogenic factors that stimulate angiogenesis. Increased vascularity also raises the likelihood of cancer cell penetration into blood vessels and/or release into the lymph or blood circulation.

   Invasion means local spread or growth into surrounding tissues. Rapid cancer cell growth increases mechanical pressure on surrounding normal tissue. This mechanical pressure causes normal tissue cells to become ischemic and necrotic, which results in low mechanical resistance around the cancer cell mass. The lower the resistance, the easier it is for cancer cells to move through the normal tissue using their inherent increased motility. Cancer cells also release a number of lytic enzymes that break down and destroy normal tissues. Again, destroyed tissue has fewer barriers and less resistance. Physiologic barriers such as dense capsules can retard but not prevent tumor cell growth and invasion. Again, local invasion increases the likelihood of cancer cell penetration into blood vessels and/or release into the lymph or blood circulation.

   Once cancer cells enter the lymph or blood circulation, they can be transported to a secondary site. Once at this distant location, they adhere to the vessel walls and eventually move into the surrounding tissue.

Cancer in Children

OBJECTIVES

After review of this chapter, the learner will be able to:

1. Describe the incidence and types of childhood cancer.

2. Discuss some of the characteristic differences in cancer between children and adults.

3. Discuss the relative importance of host, genetic, and environmental factors in the occurrence, identification, and treatment of childhood cancer.

4. Discuss the prognosis in childhood cancer.

LECTURE OUTLINE	INSTRUCTOR'S NOTES

Incidence and types of childhood cancer
Etiology
    Genetic factors
    Environmental factors
Prognosis

DIFFICULT CONCEPTS

Embryonic tumors may be a new concept to students. Thier intrauterine origin may not have been presented in previous coursework. Stressing the progress in treatments and the prognosis in childhood cancer will help students, who have recently left childhood, accept this concept.

CRITICAL THINKING

1. What are the risk factors for developing a childhood cancer?

Answer: Unlike adults, most children diagnosed with cancer do not demonstrate any predisposing environmental or host factors. Genetic factors may involve chromosome abberations, single gene defects or chromosome abnormalties. Few childhood cancers share a strong association with environmental factors. Childhood exposure to some drugs, ionizing radiation, and viruses have been implicated as risk factors. Drugs include: D.E.S., anabolic steroids, cytotoxic agents, and immunosuppressive agents.

Structure and Function of the Neurologic System

OBJECTIVES

After review of this chapter, the learner will be able to:

1. List the structures contained within the central nervous system.

2. Identify the functional divisions of the nervous system.

3. Diagram a neuron and discuss the variants of polarity and myelination.

4. Discuss synaptic transmission of impulses by neurotransmitters including the regulation mechanisms of the process.

5. Develop a chart describing the three regions of the brain with focus on location, discrete structures, function, and outputs.

6. Define a reflex arc and give an example.

7. Diagram the circulation of blood and cerebrospinal fluid through the brain and spinal cord.

8. Describe the sensory and motor functions of the peripheral nervous system.

9. Discuss the effects of sympathetic and parasympathetic stimulation on the body systems.

10. Describe tests performed to assess the function and integrity of the nervous system.

LECTURE OUTLINE	INSTRUCTOR'S NOTES

Overview and Organization of the Nervous System
Cells of the Nervous System
    The neuron
    Neuroglia and Schwann cells
    Nerve injury and regeneration
The Nerve Impulse
    Synapses
    Neurotransmitters
The Central Nervous System
    The brain
        Forebrain
        Midbrain
        Hindbrain
    The spinal cord
    Motor pathways
    Sensory pathways
    Protective structures of the central nervous system
        Cranium
        Meninges

LECTURE OUTLINE	**INSTRUCTOR'S NOTES**

            Cerebrospinal fluid and the ventricular system
            Vertebral column
       Blood supply of the central nervous system
            Blood supply to the brain
            Blood-brain barrier
            Blood supply to the spinal cord
The Peripheral Nervous System
The Autonomic Nervous System
       Anatomy of the sympathetic nervous system
       Anatomy of the parasympathetic nervous system
       Neurotransmitters and neuroreceptors
       Functions of the autonomic nervous system
Aging and the Nervous System

DIFFICULT CONCEPTS

Organization of the Nervous System

Thibodeau and Patton's analogy of telephone engineering as a model for beginning a study of the nervous system is well liked. When a telephone engineer first learns about telephone systems, the easy concept of a 2-telephone system is reviewed. Only later are more complex systems studied, such as switching systems and satellite relays. Likewise, the study of the nervous system begins with the simplest notion, the neuron, and the simplest pathway, the reflex arc. Later, more complexity (topics such as contralateral control, "switching" in the cerebrum, or cerebral impulses controlling function in the opposite side of the body) will be introduced.

Tracts Within the Central Nervous System

Students sometimes have difficulty with the concept of tracts within the central nervous system. An example of a telephone cable can be used as a model for clarification. The cable is composed of bundles of wire within an insulating tube. Each wire within the bundle may terminate at a different location, similar to distribution of a nerve tract from the brain to different points in the body (motor tracts) or from different points in the body to the brain (sensory fiber tracts).

Neurotransmitters and Neuroreceptors

Students often have difficulty understanding how one neurotransmitter can have different effects in different postsynaptic cells. This problem is easily overcome by emphasizing the point that the type of receptor mediates the postsynaptic effects. One type of neurotransmitter can bind to several types of receptors in the postsynaptic plasma membrane, each type producing different effects when stimulated. Examples that can be used include the sympathetic nervous system with the neurotransmitter norepinephrine and alpha and beta receptors. Also point out the exceptions, e.g., beta receptors in the conductive tissues of the heart mimic alpha effects (see Table 11-7). If the key-in-a-lock analogy is used, remind students that in some automobiles, one key can be used to open both the car's door and its trunk. It's the receptor (the lock) that is different, not the transmitter (the key).

Blood-Brain Barrier

The capillary walls of the brain serve as a barrier for the movement of selected chemicals and molecules from the blood to the brain tissue. An example of a set of sieves with different gauges of mesh helps to illustrate how some substances are allowed to pass through and others are not, depending on the composition and size of the substance in relation to the mesh size of the sieve.

The Cranial Nerves

The traditional pneumonics work well for learning the names, numbers, and types (motor, sensory, mixed) of the cranial nerves. The first letters of the following words are the first letters of the names of the cranial nerves, in the correct order: **O**n **O**lympus' **T**owering **T**ops, a **F**inn and **G**erman **V**iewed **S**ome **H**ops. The functional classification of each cranial nerve can be remembered using this sentence: **S**ome **S**ay **M**arry **M**oney, **B**ut **M**y **B**rothers **S**ay **B**ad **B**usiness, **M**arrying **M**oney. "S" indicates sensory, "M" indicates motor, and "B" indicates both sensory and motor (mixed).

CRITICAL THINKING

1. John, age 17, arrives unconscious following a motor vehicle accident. When his reflexes are tested, they are normal. What does this tell you about the extent of his brain injury? Why?

   Answer: Nothing. The simple reflex arc involves only the spinal cord. The brain is not involved in simple reflex arcs. Thus, the extent of the brain injury cannot be assessed by reflex testing.

Pain, Temperature, Sleep, and Sensory Function

OBJECTIVES

After review of this chapter, the learner will be able to:

1. Describe the major theories of pain: the specificity theory, the intensity theory, the gate control theory, and the pattern theory.

2. Differentiate between acute and chronic pain.

3. Describe the process of normal thermoregulation.

4. Discuss the effects of the three major alterations in body temperature: fever, hyperthermia, and hypothermia.

5. Identify and discuss the normal sleep cycle.

6. Describe the types of sleep disorders and give an example of each.

7. Describe the common ocular pathophysiologies, including causation, manifestations, and complications.

8. Differentiate between conductive and sensorineural hearing losses.

9. Describe alterations in smell and taste with causation and effect.

10. Define normal proprioception and identify the effects of altered proprioception.

LECTURE OUTLINE	INSTRUCTOR'S NOTES

Pain
   The experience of pain
      Somatogenic versus psychogenic pain
      Acute versus chronic pain
      Pain threshold and pain tolerance
   Neuroanatomy of pain
      The role of the afferent and efferent pathways
   Neurophysiology of pain
      Neuromodulation
   Clinical manifestations of pain
Temperature Regulation
   Hypothalamic control of temperature
      Mechanisms of heat production and loss
      Mechanisms of heat conservation
   Temperature regulation in infants and elderly
   Pathogenesis of fever
   Benefits of fever
   Disorders of temperature regulation
      Hyperthermia
      Hypothermia

LECTURE OUTLINE	INSTRUCTOR'S NOTES

Trauma
Sleep
  Sleep disorders
    Disorders of initiating sleep: insomnia
    Disorders of excessive somnolence
    Disorders of the sleep-wake schedule
    Dysfunctions of sleep, sleep stages, or partial
      arousals
The Special Senses
  Vision
    The eye and its external structures
    Visual dysfunction
    External eye structure disorders
  Hearing
    The normal ear
    Auditory dysfunction
    Ear infections
  Olfaction and taste
    Olfactory and taste dysfunctions
Somatosensory Function
  Touch
  Proprioception

DIFFICULT CONCEPTS

Function of the Vestibular Organs of the Ear

    Students often have difficulty understanding how equilibrium changes are detected by the endolymph in the semicircular canals. The faculty in the Physiology Department at the University of Utah have used tubular balloons partially filled with water as an effective example. Two balloons are arranged horizontally around the head; two other balloons extend vertically from the front to the back of the head and one obliquely from front to back. As the head moves in different planes, students can observe the motion of the fluid in the balloons as an analogy to the endolymph movement in the semicircular canals.

CRITICAL THINKING

1. Mr. Bowers has a temperature of 101 degrees. His physician chooses not to treat the temperature unless it rises above 103 degrees. Why?

   Answer: Fever production helps to kill or prevent the replication of many microorganisms by decreasing serum iron, zinc, and copper needed for bacterial replication and causing lysosomal breakdown and autodestruction of cells. Fever enhances the body's immune response to microorganisms by increasing the motility of PMNs, intensifying phagocytosis, increasing lymphocytic transformation, and augmenting the production of antiviral interferon.

2. Ms. Windsong suffered a head injury from a motor vehicle accident. She injured her right ear, her right occipital lobe, her right temporal lobe, and parts of her diencephalon. She has the following sensory deficits: hyposmia, inability to hear high-frequency sounds, and bilaeral left hemianopia. Explain what these sensory deficits are and why they occurred.

   Answer: All of Ms. Windsong's injuries occurred because of her head and ear injuries. Hyposmia is a decrease in smell that results from damage to one of her olfactory nerve tracts located near the diencephalon and ear. Her inability to hear high-frequency sounds is a result of the loss of auditory neurons in the spiral ganglia of the organ of Corti in her right ear. Bilateral left hemianopia results from injury to the right optic nerve tract. She is blind in her right eye's lateral (outer) field and her left eye's medial field. The optic nerve injury is located proximal to the optic chiasm, affecting her entire right optic tract.

Concepts of Neurologic Dysfunction

OBJECTIVES

After review of this chapter, the learner will be able to:

1. Identify the major causes of altered levels of arousal with differentiating manifestations and short-term and long-term effects.

2. Identify the areas of the brain and pathophysiologic theories associated with disorders of cognition.

3. Compare and contrast the major motor syndromes: CNS motor, motor unit, pyramidal, extrapyramidal, cerebellar, and upper and lower motor neuron.

4. Demonstrate and describe posturing responses.

5. Differentiate between neuropathies and myopathies.

6. Identify the areas of the brain damaged when the manifestations are alterations in emotions and behaviors.

7. Identify the major cerebral function deficits from cognitive descriptions of behaviors.

8. Compare and contrast the various forms of dysphasia.

9. List the causes of cerebral edema and give examples of pathophysiology producing each.

10. Describe the mechanisms and manifestations of the herniation syndromes.

LECTURE OUTLINE	INSTRUCTOR'S NOTES

Alterations in Cognitive Systems
    Alterations in arousal (coma)
        Level of consciousness
        Pattern of breathing
        Vomiting
        Pupillary changes
        Oculomotor responses
        Motor responses
        Outcomes
        Seizures
    Cognitive disorders
        Agnosia
        Dysphasia
        Acute confusional states
        Dementia
Alterations in Cerebral Homeostasis
    Increased intracranial pressure
    Cerebral edema
    Hydrocephalus

LECTURE OUTLINE	INSTRUCTOR'S NOTES

Alterations in Motor Function
    Alterations in muscle tone
        Hypotonia
        Hypertonia
    Alterations in movement
        Hyperkinesia
        Hypokinesia
    Alterations in complex motor performance
        Disorders of posture (stance)
        Disorders of gait
        Disorders of expression
    Extrapyramidal motor syndromes
        Basal ganglia motor syndromes
        Cerebellar motor syndromes

DIFFICULT CONCEPTS

The Central Nervous System

    Pathophysiologies of the central nervous system are very difficult for students to comprehend. The content in Chapter 13 has been divided into sections that facilitate a progressive understanding of this information. Disturbances of cognition are differentiated into alterations in arousal, including types of coma and alterations of thought. The summaries included in Tables 13-1 and 13-2 assist students to order the mechanisms and manifestations characterizing types of coma. Levels of coma or arousal are differentiated in Table 13-3 and illustrate progressive stages leading to coma.

Arousal and Cognition

    Another confusing task is differentiating alterations in arousal from alterations in cognition. A comparison of Tables 13-3 and 13-11 can assist students to begin to understand these differences.

Hierarchical Structures

    The idea that symptoms can be related to alterations in hierarchical structures can be illustrated by changes in breathing patterns, as presented in Table 13-4, or changes in motor function considering pyramidal, extrapyramidal, and motor unit dysfunction (Figure 13-11 and Tables 13-17 and 13-18). Success in understanding the complexities of neurologic dysfunction requires that students be able to associate changes in structure with changes in function.

CRITICAL THINKING

1. Ms. Spinosa has increased intracranial pressure of 30 mm Hg as a result of a massive closed head injury. Explain the process of increasing intracranial pressure and discuss possible complications if the pressure is not decreased.

   Answer: Supratentorial processes that cause a decreased level of consciousness are caused by injury somewhere above the tentorium. In this case, Ms. Spinosa suffered diffuse bilateral cortical dysfunction that caused widespread injury throughout the cerebral cortex and in the subcortical white matter. In Ms. Spinosa's injury, her intracranial pressure increased from a normal 5-15 mm Hg to 30 mm Hg because of intracerebral hemorrhage or edema. The brain tissue is displaced and the blood vessels are distorted.

   In Stage 1, the increasing pressure forces the cerebrospinal fluid (CSF) out of the cranial vault, compresses the intracranial veins, and increases venous vasoconstriction. Often intracranial pressure will not change during this stage because blood volume and CSF volumes are reduced. Stage 2 occurs when pressure is not relieved. Arterial blood vessels constrict, compromising oxygen supply. The systemic arterial system will also constrict in order to increase BP. The elevated systemic BP is an attempt to overcome the intracranial pressure.

   When intracranial pressure increases and approaches arterial pressure, Stage 3 intracranial hypertension occurs. During this stage, tissue hypoxia, hypercapnia, and acidosis occur. Autoregulation of blood vessel diameter is lost. Hypercapnia causes local vasodilation with subsequent increasing capillary permeability. As increasing cerebral edema occurs, intracranial pressure increases. Small changes in volume cause dramatic increases in pressure with decreased cerebral perfusion pressure.

   Stage 4 is characterized by herniation of the brain from the compartment of greater pressure to one of lower pressure. In Ms. Spinosa's case, the brain herniated downward (supratentorial herniation), causing central or uncal herniation. Blood supply and brain tissue is markedly compromised or completely cut off, causing further ischemia, hypoxia, and hemorrhage in the herniated portion of the brain. When mean systolic pressure equals intracranial pressure, blood flow to the brain stops.

2. Injury to your extrapyramidal motor system does not cause paralysis of voluntary movement and general spasticity. Explain why and discuss the major motor symptoms seen in extrapyramidal motor disorders.

   Answer: The extrapyramidal motor system includes all motor pathways in the brain and brain stem that are not part of the corticospinal or pyramidal motor pathways. This system includes the basal ganglia, reticular formation, and parts of the cerebellum. Disorders are classified as either basal ganglia motor or cerebellar motor syndromes. Both are characterized by little or no paralysis of voluntary movement; normal or slightly increased tendon reflexes; presence of tremor, chorea, athetosis or dystonia; and rigidity or intermittent rigidity. Muscle tone and equilibrium are also affected.

Alterations of Neurologic Function

OBJECTIVES

After review of this chapter, the learner will be able to:

1. Define the different types of head injury with examples of the type of force needed to produce each.

2. Discuss the manifestations of complete and partial spinal cord injuries in both the acute and rehabilitative phases.

3. Identify known causes of low back pain.

4. Describe the pathophysiologies producing interruption to cerebral vascular flow with reference to location, manifestations, and rehabilitation potential.

5. Discuss the cellular pathophysiology, manifestations, and treatment of the central nervous system tumors.

6. Describe infectious processes occurring in the central nervous system.

7. Identify the diseases of basal ganglia degeneration and describe the manifestations, treatment, and prognosis of each.

8. Describe the different syndromes that determine the initial manifestations of multiple sclerosis.

9. Differentiate between upper and lower motor neuron diseases.

LECTURE OUTLINE	INSTRUCTOR'S NOTES

Central Nervous System (CNS) Disorders
    Trauma
        Head trauma
        Spinal cord trauma
        Low back pain
        Herniated intervertebral disk
    Cerebrovascular disorders
        Cerebrovascular accidents
        Arteriovenous malformation
        Subarachnoid hemorrhage
    Infection and inflammation of the central nervous
        system
        Meningitis
        Abscess
        Encephalitis
        Neurologic complications of AIDS
    Degenerative diseases

LECTURE OUTLINE	INSTRUCTOR'S NOTES

Alzheimer diseases
Pick disease
Parkinson disease
Huntington disease
Multiple sclerosis
Amyotrophic lateral sclerosis
Peripheral Nervous System and Neuromuscular Junction
Disorders
Peripheral nervous system disorders
Neuromuscular junction disorders
Myasthenia gravis
Myopathies
Tumors of the Central Nervous System
Cranial tumors
Spinal cord tumors

DIFFICULT CONCEPTS

Autonomic Hyperreflexia

This concept is difficult because of a necessary prerequisite understanding of the sympathetic, parasympathetic, spinothalamic, and corticospinal tracts; cranial nerve function; and baroreceptor function. It is the interaction among these pathways that causes the complexity. Figure 14-12 illustrates the normal response pathway: visceral distention —> spinothalamic tracts —> brain interpretation of sensory input —> corticospinal tracts —> motor output. Autonomic dysreflexia: visceral distention —> spinothalamic tract to level of lesion —> reflex stimulus to sympathetic outflow —> increased blood pressure stimulates carotid sinus receptors —> cranial nerve, vagus nerve stimulation —> bradycardia —> autonomic response to hypertension. Students seem to understand the process if the normal response pathway is also reviewed.

Degenerative Diseases: Parkinson Disease, Huntington Disease, and Multiple Sclerosis

The most difficult aspect of the degenerative neurologic diseases is understanding where in the nervous system they originate. Much confusion with this content is related to a lack of understanding of normal nervous system anatomy. It is, therefore, helpful to use slides of normal anatomy to demonstrate, for example, the basal ganglia, substantia nigra, and central nervous system myelin.

CRITICAL THINKING

1. Two individuals come to the emergency room with head injuries. One, age 25, has just been in a motor vehicle accident (MVA) and has a temporal lobe injury. The other, age 65, has increasing confusion following a fall that happened earlier in the week. How could you clinically differentiate between the individual with the extradural hematoma and the individual with the subdural hematoma? Which one of these individuals requires priority surgical treatment?

   Answer: An extradural hematoma or epidural hemorrhage is a rapidly accumulating arterial bleed occurring between the skull and dura mater. Injuries to the temporal lobe are often associated with extradural hematomas because the middle meningeal artery runs in a groove on the surface before entering the skull. Extradural hematomas are most commonly caused by MVAs and are frequently associated with temporal lobe injuries. An epidural hemorrhage is characterized by loss of consciousness at the time of injury followed by a lucid period. Within a few hours, symptoms will progress from severe headache, vomiting, and drowsiness to confusion, seizures, ipsilateral pupillary dilatation, and contralateral hemiparesis. An extradural hematoma is always a medical emergency, so the individual in the MVA would require priority surgical treatment.

   A subdural hematoma is a venous bleed occurring between the dura mater and the arachnoid mater. Subdural bleeds occur more slowly, ranging from hours to weeks. The range in the delay depends on how many veins were torn, the size of the epidural space, and the amount of compression on the bleeding veins. Once a vein is torn, it will bleed and compress the brain. As intracranial pressure increases, the bleeding veins will be compressed, slowing the amount of bleeding. A subdural hematoma can also be caused in a motor vehicle accident but is commonly the result of falls in the elderly. In the elderly, the symptoms of a subdural hematoma vary from a chronic headache and drowsiness to slowed cognition, confusion, progressive dementia, and paratonia (generalized rigidity). A subdural hematoma will require surgery to evacuate the clot but would not take priority over the individual with the extradural hematoma.

2. Ms. Evans has a flexion injury with resultant incomplete spinal cord transection at level C4-5. What symptoms would you expect Ms. Evans to have 1 month after her injury?

   Answer: She would have Brown-Sequard syndrome with (1) ipsilateral paralysis below C4-5 with return of Babinski reflexes and ankle and knee reflexes; (2) ipsilateral loss of touch, pressure, vibration, and proprioception with possible paresthesia below the level of transection; and (3) contralateral loss of pain and temperature. She may experience autonomic hyperreflexia (dysreflexia). She may also have some reappearance of reflex defecation and reflex urination.

Alterations of Neurologic Function in Children

OBJECTIVES

After review of this chapter, the learner will be able to:

1. Describe the six stages of development of the nervous system and give specific examples of disorders resulting from abnormal or delayed maturation of the system.

2. Identify four major congenital abnormalities of the central nervous system and discuss the manifestations, treatment, and prognosis of each.

3. Discuss the occurrence and causes of seizure disorders in childhood with a focus on differential manifestations and treatment from that of adults.

4. Describe the cellular findings, manifestations, risk factors, and outcomes in Reye syndrome.

5. Describe the differences in central nervous system tumors in children and adults.

6. Identify the common types of central nervous system tumors found in children.

LECTURE OUTLINE	INSTRUCTOR'S NOTES

Normal Growth and Development of the Nervous
    System
Structural Malformations
    Defects of neural tube closure
    Malformations of the axial skeleton
        Spina bifida occulta
        Cranial deformities
Encephalopathies
    Static encephalopathies
Inherited Metabolic Disorders of the CNS
    Defects in amino acid metabolism
    Defects in lipid metabolism
Seizure Disorders
    Epilepsy
Acute Encephalopathies
    Reye syndrome
    Intoxications of the CNS
    Meningitis
Human Immunodeficiency Virus (HIV) and CNS
Involvement

LECTURE OUTLINE	INSTRUCTOR'S NOTES

Tumors
    Brain tumors
    Embryonal tumors
        Neuroblastoma
        Retinoblastoma

DIFFICULT CONCEPTS

Types of Possible Disorders

Students can more easily grasp the alterations of neurologic function in children if they have an overall conceptual orientation to the types of possible disorders; for example, congenital malformations, encephalopathies, trauma, infections, tumors, and vascular disorders. Students can then work in small groups to develop a set of taxonomies within each category to further refine their understanding. For example, seizure disorders are classified as partial, generalized, or unclassified and can be partial or complete. With this level of conceptual structure, etiologies and clinical manifestations can then be established. A similar process can be used for approaching childhood brain tumors. Tumors are either supratentorial or infratentorial, with most in children being the latter. Cell types can then be identified and classified as fast or slow growing. From this information, students have a basis for beginning to understand the clinical manifestations of the different tumors.

CRITICAL THINKING

1. Explain the difference between brain tumors found in children and brain tumors found in adults.

   Answer: Most brain tumors (70%) found in children are infratentorial, in the posterior third of the brain. Theories suggest that genetic factors may be involved in the development of childhood brain tumors, with some increased frequency within families. Another theory suggests that these tumors are of embryonic origin, where embryonic cells are misplaced and later replicate in their embryonic form. The most frequent type of childhood brain tumor is cerebellar astrocytoma, which is a slow growing tumor.

   Most brain tumors (70%) found in adults are supratentorial, in the anterior two-thirds of the brain. In adults, the most common type of tumor is glioblastoma multiforme, which is a rapidly growing, highly malignant tumor located predominantly in the cerebral hemispheres.

2. Differentiate between the clinical findings commonly associated with congenital hydrocephalus that occurs in infancy and those commonly associated with hydrocephalus that occurs in older children.

   Answer: The infant with congenital hydrocephalus would not exhibit early signs of increasing intracranial pressure because of her flexible skull. At birth, she either may be asymptomatic or may have an abnormally enlarged head. As the infant grows, her skull grows out of proportion to both her face and body, becoming abnormally large. She has enlarged fontanelles and separated cranial sutures. Her scalp veins are prominent and her scalp skin is thin. Her skull resonates when tapped; this is called Macewen or "cracked-pot" sign. Her eyes widen with her sclera visible (called "sunset sign"). She may have difficulty holding her head upright. Without treatment, she may develop an abnormal cry and have compression of the optic nerves.

   The older child who develops hydrocephalus does not have an enlarged head because the cranial sutures are fixed and the skull is rigid. She would develop signs of increasing intracranial pressure with headache.

Mechanisms of Hormonal Regulation

OBJECTIVES

After review of this chapter, the learner will be able to:

1. Identify the functions of the endocrine system.

2. Discuss the regulation of hormone secretion by positive and negative feedback loops.

3. Discuss cellular mechanisms of hormone action.

4. Identify the hormones of the anterior pituitary (including the appropriate releasing factor), stimulating hormones, target hormones, and target tissues, including normal outcomes.

5. Describe the hormones of the posterior pituitary and their actions.

6. Discuss the similarities and differences between the thyroid hormones T3, T4, and calcitonin.

7. Identify the hormones secreted by the alpha, beta, and delta cells of the pancreas.

8. Identify the adrenocortical and medullary hormones with reference to structure, function, and regulation of secretion by the body systems.

LECTURE OUTLINE	INSTRUCTOR'S NOTES

Mechanisms of Hormonal Regulation
    Regulation of hormone release
    Hormone transport
    Mechanisms of hormone action
        Hormone receptors
        First and second messengers
        Steroid (lipid-soluble) hormone receptors
Structure and Function of the Endocrine Glands
    Hypothalamic-pituitary system
        Anterior pituitary
        Posterior pituitary
    Thyroid and parathyroid glands
        Thyroid gland
        Parathyroid glands
    Endocrine pancreas
        Insulin
        Amylin
        Glucagon
        Somatostatin

LECTURE OUTLINE	INSTRUCTOR'S NOTES

Adrenal glands
    Adrenal cortex
    Adrenal medulla
Neuroendocrine response to stressors

DIFFICULT CONCEPTS

Neuroendocrine Interrelationships

Interactions between the endocrine and nervous systems coordinate important integrative responses the body must make to changes occurring in the internal and external environment. Examples that assist student understanding include decreases in blood glucose levels and dehydration states. When there is a decrease in blood glucose, the endocrine system responds with hormones from the anterior pituitary (ACTH and GH), pancreas (glucagon), adrenal medulla (epinephrine and norepinephrine), and adrenal cortex (cortisol). The nervous system responds with neurohormones from the hypothalamus and sympathetic nervous system. All secretions combine to act on the liver, muscle, and adipose tissue to restore blood glucose levels. In dehydration states, blood volume will decrease, which is sensed by vascular baroreceptors, the cardiac atria, the kidney, and the brain. The sympathetic nervous system is activated, a neurohormone is released from the posterior pituitary (ADH), and hormones are released from the cardiac atria (atrial natriuretic hormone), adrenal medulla (aldosterone), adrenal cortex (cortisol), and kidneys (renin), which act on blood vessels and the kidneys to restore blood volume.

Hormone Receptor Action

The example of a key in a lock as a model of hormone receptor action illustrates the different effects produced by different hormone receptor interactions. For example, one key in a lock may open the car door, another key in the lock may turn on the house security system.

Second Messenger Hypothesis

The idea of a second messenger can often be confusing to beginning students. The operation of a telephone answering machine demonstrates the second messenger mechanism. The first message is the call (hormone) which is received by the answering machine (cell membrane). The recording of the message by the answering machine is the second messenger (C-AMP or calcium) which directs the recipient (cell) with information. The recipient (cell) receives the message from the answering machine and carries out the message, such as going to the store to buy milk. The process is the person going to the store to buy milk. The outcome, the person buying milk, represents the effect of the first messenger which is made possible by the second messenger.

CRITICAL THINKING

1. Describe the physiologic processess involved in ADH secretion.

   Answer: The secretion of ADH is primarily by osmoreceptors in the hypothymus, but also by baroreceptors in the left atrium, the carotids, and the aortic arches. The posterior pituitary releases ADH. Mediators are cholinergic and adrenergic neurotransmitters. ADH secretion is increased by changes in intravascular volume and decreased plasma. Osmolality, stress, trauma, pain, exercise, nausea, nicotine, exposure to heat, and drugs can also increase secretion. Decreased plasma osmolality, increased intravascular volume, hypertension, and alcohol ingestion decreases ADH secretion.

Alterations of Hormonal Regulation

OBJECTIVES

After review of this chapter, the learner will be able to:

1. Identify the mechanisms of hormonal dysfunction.

2. Compare SIADH and diabetes insipidus including causative factors, cellular pathophysiology, manifestations, treatment, and prognosis.

3. Discuss the causes of hyper- and hypopituitarism with consideration of the populations at highest risk for the development of the disoders.

4. Explain the progression of hyperthyroidism through Graves disease and thyroid storm with cellular changes, manifestations, treatments, and complications.

5. Discuss the causes, treatment options, and outcomes for disorders producing hypothyroidism.

6. Differentiate between primary, secondary, and tertiary hyperparathyroidism.

7. Discuss the similarities and differences in the etiology and pathophysiology of insulin dependent and noninsulin-dependent diabetes mellitus.

8. Describe the acute complications of diabetes mellitus with a focus on differential detection and treatment.

9. List the chronic complications of diabetes mellitus and discuss how good control of blood sugar limits the cellular degeneration in each instance.

10. Describe tumors of the adrena medulla.

LECTURE OUTLINE	INSTRUCTOR'S NOTES

Mechanisms of Hormonal Alterations
Alterations of the Hypothalamic-Pituitary System
    Diseases of the posterior pituitary
        Syndrome of inappropriate antidiuretic
            hormone secretion
        Diabetes insipidus
    Diseases of the anterior pituitary
        Hypopituitarism
        Hyperpituitarism: primary adenoma
        Hypersecretion of growth hormone:
            acromegaly
Alterations of Thyroid Function
    Thyrotoxicosis
        Course of thyrotoxicosis
        Hyperthyroid conditions

LECTURE OUTLINE	INSTRUCTOR'S NOTES

Hypothyroidism
    Hypothyroid conditions
    Thyroid carcinoma
Alterations of Parathyroid Function
    Hyperparathyroidism
    Hypoparathyroidism
Dysfunction of the Endocrine Pancreas: Diabetes
    Mellitus
    Types of diabetes mellitus
        Type 1 diabetes mellitus
        Type 2 diabetes mellitus
        Gestational diabetes
    Acute complications of diabetes mellitus
    Chronic complications of diabetes mellitus
        Hyperglycemia and nonenzymatic glycosylation
        Hyperglycemia and polyol pathway
        Protein kinase C
        Diabetic neuropathies
        Microvascular disease
        Macrovascular disease
        Infection
Alterations of Adrenal Function
    Disorders of the adrenal cortex
        Hypercortical function (Cushing disease,
            Cushing syndrome)
        Congenital adrenal hyperplasia
        Hyperaldosteronism
        Hypersecretion of adrenal androgens and
            estrogens
        Hypocortical functioning
    Disorders of the adrenal medulla
        Tumors of the adrenal medulla

DIFFICULT CONCEPTS

Diabetes Mellitus

    The multiple metabolic consequences of diabetes mellitus contribute to complexity and confusion in learning about this disease. Comparing diabetes mellitus to long-term starvation provides some clarification. In long-term starvation states there is not access to adequate carbohydrates from dietary sources. The body consumes its immediate fuel resource glycogen and turns to metabolism of fats and later proteins, contributing to a state of ketoacidosis and weight loss. Although there is not hyperglycemia in starvation, the inadequate access to glucose by cells is similar to lack of cellular glucose due to altered insulin sources or utilization, as occurs in diabetes mellitus. In both states, ketoacidosis is related to excess utilization of fat and protein as a source of energy.

Systemic Manifestations of Endocrine Disorders

    Alterations of specific endocrine glands result in function changes in multiple organs. The multiple changes may initially be difficult for students to comprehend because hormones are often described as having specific target cells or tissues. Assisting students to learn that target cells for a particular hormone may be located in several different organs and that alterations in specific organs often lead to compensatory changes in other organs will facilitate understanding of multiple organ symptoms.

CRITICAL THINKING

1. Mr. Metzner has polyuria with a urine volume of 8 L/day. His urine specific gravity is 1.02. His serum sodium (Na⁺) is 150, and his plasma osmolality is 300 mOsm/kg. He is always asking for more cold liquids to drink. What type of hormonal alteration is Mr. Metzner exhibiting? What are some possible causes of this alteration?

   Answer: Mr. Metzner has diabetes insipidus, which has three forms: neurogenic, nephrogenic, and psychogenic. The neurogenic form is caused by a hypothalamic, infundibular stem, or posterior pituitary problem that decreases or inhibits ADH synthesis, transport, or release. This may be caused by pituitary tumors, brain tumors, infections, immunologic problems, or thrombotic problems.

   The nephrogenic form of diabetes insipidus may be acquired, permanent, or reversible. It is caused by renal tubule insensitivity to ADH. In this form, the amounts of ADH are normal, but the tubules are no longer able to respond to the hormone. Examples of renal problems that can lead to diabetes insipidus include pyelonephritis, amyloidosis, destructive uropathies, and polycystic disease. It may also be the result of anesthetic drug use or the use of lithium carbonate.

   The psychogenic form of diabetes insipidus is caused by compulsive water drinking by individuals with psychiatric disorders. In this form, the individual has periodic polyuria, high urine volume, and plasma osmolarity of less than 285 mOsm/kg.

2. Analyze the difference in pathophysiology between type 1 diabetes mellitus and type 2 diabetes mellitus.

   Answer: In type 1 diabetes mellitus, the beta cells in the islets of Langerhans are destroyed. This destruction is progressive and associated with the presence of IgG islet cell antibodies (ICA), suggesting an autoimmune process. At the clinical onset of the disease, 80% to 90% of all insulin-secreting beta cells in the islets of Langerhans are destroyed, leaving a small number of little, atrophic, and fibrotic cells left. Within one year, all remaining cells are destroyed. Coinciding with beta cell destruction, there is abnormal alpha cell function resulting in excess glucagon production. Therefore, the functional deficit in type 1 diabetes mellitus is both a lack of insulin production and an excess of glucagon production.

   The cause of this destructive process has been theorized to include a viral disease, an immune reaction, or inherited susceptibility combined with environmental factors. In all likelihood, type 1 diabetes mellitus may be a combination of all of these factors. The autoimmune process may be triggered by viral infection such as coxsackie B4 virus or mumps. This is highly supported by the increased incidence of type 1 diabetes in the fall and winter in the northern hemisphere when there are increased viral infections. Type 1 diabetes mellitus may also be linked genetically. There is an association between type 1 and HLA-D and HLA-DR alleles—particularly HLA-DR3 and HLA-DR4.

   In type 2 diabetes mellitus, the cellular changes are more nonspecific. Islet cells are progressively replaced with hyalin tissue, an albuminoid substance, leaving a decrease in the size and number of beta cells. There is also fatty infiltration in both the liver and pancreas, causing increased tissue size and the presence of glycogen vacuoles. However, the ratio of alpha to beta cells in the pancreas is normal and the plasma and pancreatic levels of insulin are not decreased. Many of these changes are similar in aging persons both with and without type 2 diabetes mellitus.

   According to the World Health Organization (WHO), the strongest risk factor for the development of type 2 diabetes mellitus is obesity. Type 2 diabetes mellitus has been theorized to include genetic susceptibility combined with obesity. The causes have been thought to involve insulin receptors in the plasma membrane and insulin resistance. One theory advocates that a decreased number of insulin receptors causes decreased insulin binding. Another theory states that intracellular events after insulin receptor binding are altered. Several theories explore the relationship between hyperinsulinemia and type 2 diabetes mellitus. One of these theories suggests that the islet cells "give out" over time in an effort to produce enough insulin to compensate for obesity. Another states that hyperinsulinemia causes cellular insulin resistance to protect against hypoglycemia. Therefore, the functional deficit in type 2 diabetes mellitus is a combination of obesity, increased insulin resistance, and an excess of glucagon production.

Structure and Function of the Hematologic System

OBJECTIVES

After review of this chapter, the learner will be able to:

1. Describe the composition of blood.

2. Discuss the structure and function of the cellular components of blood.

3. Identify the roles of the mononuclear phagocyte system.

4. Describe the differentiation of the cellular components of blood from common stem cells.

5. Discuss the role of the colony stimulating factors (CSFs), identifying the specific CSFs for neutrophils, macrophages, and erythrocytes.

6. Identify the vitamins and hormones essential to the generation and maturation of blood cells.

7. Describe the four stages of the hemostatic mechanism.

8. Describe the process of clot dissolution.

LECTURE OUTLINE	INSTRUCTOR'S NOTES

Components of the Hematologic System
  Composition of the blood
    Plasma and plasma proteins
    Cellular components of the blood
  Lymphoid organs
    Spleen
    Lymph nodes
  The mononuclear phagocyte sytem (MPS)
Development of Blood Cells
  Hematopoiesis
    Stem cell system
    Clinical uses of CSFs
    Bone marrow
  Development of erythrocytes
    Hemoglobin synthesis
    Nutritional requirements for erythropoiesis
    Iron cycle
    Regulation of erythropoiesis
    Normal destruction of senescent erythrocytes
  Development of leukocytes
  Development of platelets

LECTURE OUTLINE	INSTRUCTOR'S NOTES

Mechanisms of Hemostasis
    Function of platelets and blood vessels
    Function of clotting factors
    Control of hemostatic mechanisms
    Retraction and lysis of blood clots

DIFFICULT CONCEPTS

Stem Cell System (Blood Cell Differentiation)

Blood cell development can be compared to the structure of the pyramids. In this hierarchical system, the earliest, most primitive ancestor (top of the pyramid) is the totipotential hematopoietic stem cell (THSC). As you descend the pyramid, it becomes larger; many more blood cells have developed from the THSC. The multiple pathways of differentiation require cytokines or hematopoietic growth factors that stimulate (broadening of the pyramid base) the proliferation of fully mature cells. Figure 18-5 visually helps students with the pyramid image.

Control of Hemostatic Mechanisms

This concept is easier to understand if students can see the normal vascular endothelium using a slide, transparency, or drawing on the board. It is important to emphasize that activation of the clotting factors, inhibition of these active clotting factors, and the production of circulating anticoagulant proteins takes place on membrane surfaces (e.g., endothelium). Showing diagrams of the endothelium while discussing the regulatory events in the clotting process helps the student to retain this important information.

CRITICAL THINKING

1. Mrs. M. is diagnosed with neutropenia (a low level of neutrophils). What problem could this create?

    Answer: Neutrophils are the chief phagocytes in early inflammation. Decreases place her at increased risk for infection and decreases her ability to fight infection.

2. Mr. S. has a platelet count of 50,000/mm^3. What problem could this cause?

    Answer: This platelet count is decreased and places him at increased risk for bleeding. Platelets are necessary for normal clotting.

Alterations of Hematologic Function

OBJECTIVES

After review of this chapter, the learner will be able to:

1. Define anemia.

2. List the various methods of classifying the anemias.

3. Describe the manifestations of anemia and discuss the pathophysiology that generates them.

4. Discuss the causes of, and treatments for, the most common type of anemia worldwide.

5. Describe the normocytic-normochromic anemias.

6. Give examples of congenital and acquired hemolytic anemias.

7. Discuss the role of leukocyte endogenous mediator in the anemia associated with chronic illness.

8. Compare the anemias.

9. Discuss polycythemia vera and its causes.

10. Describe the multiple system manifestations of polycythemia vera related to the increased viscosity and volume of blood.

11. Classify leukemia as related to maturity of the cells and appearance of the total leukocyte count and differential.

12. Differentiate the leukemias by manifestations, treatment options, and prognosis.

13. Describe the manifestations of infectious mononucleosis, with attention to the complications for other systems from the infection.

14. Discuss Hodgkin and non-Hodgkin lymphomas, with a focus on differential diagnosis, manifestations, treatment, and prognosis.

15. Identify the causes of splenomegaly.

16. Identify the causes of thrombocytopenia.

17. Discuss the pathophysiology of disseminated intravascular coagulation.

18. Discuss the prethrombotic conditions that predispose an individual to the development of thrombi.

LECTURE OUTLINE

INSTRUCTOR'S NOTES

Alteration of erythrocyte function
    Classification of anemias
    Clinical manifestations of anemias
    Macrocytic-normochromic anemias
        Pernicious anemia
        Folate deficiency anemia
    Microcytic-hypochromic anemias
        Iron deficiency anemia
        Sideroblastic anemia
    Normocytic-normochromic anemias
Myeloproliferative Red Cell Disorders
    (Polycythemia Vera)
Alterations of Leukocyte Function
    Quantitative alterations of leukocytes
        Granulocytes and monocytes
        Lymphocytes
    Infectious mononucleosis
    Leukemias
        Acute leukemias
        Chronic leukemias
    Multiple myeloma
Alterations in Lymphoid Function
    Lymphadenopathy
    Malignant lymphomas
        Hodgkin disease
        Non-Hodgkin lymphoma
        Burkitt lymphoma
Alterations of Splenic Function
Alterations of Platelets and Coagulation
    Disorders of platelet function
        Thrombocytopenia
        Thrombocythemia
    Alterations of platelet function
    Disorders of coagulation
        Impaired hemostasis
        Consumptive thrombohemorrhagic disorders

DIFFICULT CONCEPTS

Classification of Anemia

Students seem to have trouble with the descriptions of anemias based on erythrocyte structure. To make this easier, show slides of each of the different size and shape erythrocytes with labels; that is, macrocytic-normochromic, microcytic-hypochromic, and normocytic-normochromic. Include examples (e.g., microcytic-hypochromic, iron-deficiency anemia, thalassemia, etc.) with each of the types.

Anemia of Chronic Inflammation

Like any disorder related to inflammation, the difficulty is understanding the cell types and interactions involved in the inflammatory response. If inflammation was reviewed early in the course, some students forget the role of cytokines, macrophages, prostaglandins, and so on. Teaching this section in a somewhat Socratic way—asking students what tumor necrosis factor, macrophages, lymphocytes, etc., do—helps involve them and makes it easier to discuss the mechanisms of anemia of chronic inflammation.

Classification of Leukemia

A difficult area for students is understanding the origin, maturation, and physiological differences among the blood cells. Because of this difficulty, students sometimes have trouble delineating among the different types of leukemia. Therefore, starting this section with Figures 19-2 helps immediately with their understanding of the classification system for leukemia. Once they visualize the type of cell affected (e.g., myeloid, granulocyte), they can better understand the point at which cell maturation is arrested and the type of clinical manifestations produced.

Clinical Manifestations of Leukemia

Because there are many manifestations of leukemia, students who are also clinicians appreciate the summary of mechanisms associated with common manifestations.

Disseminated Intravascular Coagulation (DIC)

Concepts difficult here are the mechanisms activating the intrinsic or extrinsic clotting cascade, fibrinolysis, kallikrein-kinin, and complement systems. All of these systems contribute to the thrombosis and hemorrhage characteristic of DIC. Once students understand how thrombin is activated, it is easier for them to understand hypoperfusion, ischemia, infarction, and necrosis as the result of circulatory deposition of thrombin. Figure 19-9 summarizes the pathogenesis of DIC.

CRITICAL THINKING

1. How does defective gastric secretion of intrinsic factor (IF) cause anemia? What is this type of anemia called and how do you get it?

   Answer: This type of megaloblastic anemia is called pernicious anemia. It is a macrocytic-normochromic anemia that is a deficiency or lack of gastric secretion of IF. Because IF is necessary for the absorption of vitamin B_{12}, a deficiency of IF results in an inability to absorb vitamin B_{12}. Vitamin B_{12} is needed for red blood cell maturation and DNA synthesis. Without vitamin B_{12}, there is ineffective erythropoiesis and early erythrocyte cell death, and the few remaining mature cells are unusually large with very small and defective nuclei. These cells have the normal amount of hemoglobin. Hemoglobin, hematocrit, and reticulocyte counts are low.

   This type of anemia can be the result of gastric surgery, chronic fundal gastritis, gastric atrophy, or a congenital cause. Those with IF in their families are more likely to develop pernicious anemia, suggesting an autosomal recessive genetic predisposition. The presence of autoantibodies against parietal cells and IF may also indicate an autoimmune component.

2. Ms. Blankenship has iron deficiency anemia. She has just had a total abdominal hysterectomy. Her postoperative hemoglobin is 8 and her hematocrit is 25. She states that she has been anemic for "years." What clinical findings are commonly associated with iron deficiency anemia?

   Answer: Ms. Blankenship may experience any of the following: fatigue, weakness, shortness of breath, tachycardia, and dizziness. Her skin, palms, conjunctivae, and mucous membranes will be pale. Her nails will be brittle, thin, or concave. Her tongue will be red and sore. The corners of her mouth will be sore and dry (angular stomatitis) and she may have difficulty swallowing. She may exhibit gastritis, neuromuscular changes, irritability, headache, numbness, tingling, and vasomotor disturbances. The elderly may also experience mental confusion, memory loss, and disorientation.

3. Analyze the pathophysiologic and epidemiologic similarities and differences between chronic granulocytic leukemia (CGL) and acute lymphoblastic leukemia (ALL).

   Answer: Both CGL and ALL are diseases of blood-forming organs causing growth of uncontrolled, undifferentiated, and immature lymphocytes (blast cells). These immature cells then circulate in the blood, infiltrating the liver, spleen, lymph nodes, and other tissue sites. The blood forming cells affected by ALL and CGL are the lymphoid stem cells. Both CGL and ALL tend to occur in families, suggesting hereditary susceptibility.

   ALL primarily affects children. It is both an accumulation and proliferation disorder in which a transformed mutation clones a line of poorly differentiated, abnormal daughter cells. These cells are unable to mature or respond to normal regulatory mechanisms. They also proliferate rapidly, which decreases or stops the proliferation of other cell lines in the bone marrow. ALL primarily affects either T-cell or B-cell lines. Anemia, thrombocytopenia, hemorrhage, and disseminated intravascular coagulation (DIC) usually accompany ALL. The gonads, bones, joints, central nervous system, kidneys, lungs, and gastrointestinal tract are the most common sites of infiltration.

   CGL primarily affects B-cells in adults. The cells in CGL are slow growing and well differentiated. In CGL, the B-cells are unable to mature and synthesize immunoglobulin. Therefore, individuals with CGL lack humoral immunity and have increased risk of infection, autoimmunity, and the development of secondary cancers. Anemia is usually mild, and hemorrhage is rare. Lymph node, liver, spleen, and salivary gland infiltration is common.

4. How can disseminated intravascular coagulation (DIC) cause ischemia, thrombosis, and bleeding?

   Answer: DIC is a cyclic disorder in which massive intravascular coagulation is triggered at the cellular level, producing microthrombi. The microthrombi block the microvascular system, using up clotting factors and platelets as well as causing widespread tissue ischemia. The development of widespread microthrombi formation at the cellular level also activates the fibrinolytic system, which attempts to rapidly lyse the clots. This process releases fibrin degradation or split products (FDP or FSP). The consumption of clotting factors and platelets, along with the rising levels of FSP, leads to inhibition of coagulation and bleeding. The bleeding with loss of vascular volume also contributes to tissue ischemia.

Alterations of Hematologic Function in Children

OBJECTIVES

After review of this chapter, the learner will be able to:

1. Describe the hemolytic diseases of newborns related to maternal-neonate blood incompatibilities.

2. Describe the genetic abnormalities producing sickle cell anemia and the thalassemias.

3. Differentiate between the inherited hemophilias and discuss treatment options and complications of the disorders.

4. Describe the acquired antibody-mediated hemorrhagic diseases of childhood.

5. Identify the childhood leukemias and discuss causation.

6. Describe the etiology, morbidity, and mortality in Hodgkin disease and non-Hodgkin lyphoma in childhood.

LECTURE OUTLINE	INSTRUCTOR'S NOTES

Disorders of Erythrocytes
    Acquired disorders
        Iron deficiency anemia
        Hemolytic disease of the newborn (HDN)
    Inherited disorders
        Sickle cell disease
        Thalassemias
Disorders of Coagulation and Platelets
    Inherited hemorrhagic disease
        Hemophilias
    Antibody-mediated hemorrhagic disease
        Idiopathic thrombocytopenic purpura
Neoplastic Disorders
    Leukemia and Lymphoma
        Leukemia
        Lymphoma
    Hodgkin Disease

DIFFICULT CONCEPTS

Hemolytic Disease in the Newborn (HDN)

Again, what is difficult for students is normal immune function; that is, what is antigenic and what is the antibody or cellular response. Drawing a pregnant woman on the board (if you're so bold), slowly going through the incompatibilities (e.g., ABO and Rh), and demonstrating what happens if anti-Rh antibodies persist in the mother's blood help students understand through visualization. Slowly defining sensitization, Rh-antigen, anti-Rh antibody, and immunoprophylaxis (Rh-immune globulin) is necessary. Sometimes student volunteers will draw the scenario on the board with other students yelling from their desks, some agreeing and others disagreeing on how to draw it.

Antibody-Mediated Hemorrhagic Disease

To understand this group of disorders, once again mastery of the immune response and the inflammatory response is necessary. If students are quite familiar with these responses, they "sail" through this group of disorders.

CRITICAL THINKING

1. An 8-year-old child is admitted with severe epistaxis. She has a generalized purple petechial rash that developed over the last 24 hours. She also has hemorrhage bullae on her gums and lips. Her parents state that "she just started to bleed before our eyes." She denies any recent falls. She states she just got over a "cold." Her lab work shows abnormal bleeding time, thrombocytopenia, normal granulocytes, and low normal hemoglobin and hematocrit. What type of disorder does this child have, and what is the pathophysiology?

   Answer: This child has acute idiopathic thrombocytopenic purpura (ITP). It is the most common purpura of childhood. It is an autoimmune disorder characterized by a loss of thrombocytes. The loss of large numbers of platelets is stimulated by IgG-type antiplatelet antibodies that bind to the plasma membranes of platelets. This large antigen-antibody complex is then attacked, sequestered, and cleared from the circulation by monocytes in the spleen and other lymph tissues. Approximately 70% of all cases of ITP occur approximately 2 weeks after a viral infection.

2. Why does dehydration, decreased pO_2, and decreased pH cause sickling in a child with hemoglobin S (HbS)?

   Answer: Children with HbS have a genetic hemoglobin mutation in which one amino acid, glutamic acid, is replaced by another amino acid, valine. When stressors such as dehydration, decreased pO_2 or decreased pH occur, a sickling cycle follows. Systemic or local decreased pO_2 (hypoxemia) causes HbS cells to form an elongated crescent shape due to reaggregation of hemoglobin into long chains. This shape causes the red blood cell membranes to become stiff, thus losing some of their capacity for active transport.

   In a hypoxemic state, sickling is further promoted in the microcirculation when hemoglobin releases oxygen to the tissues, and the microcirculation is clogged by sickled cells. This results in further stagnation and hypoxemia. Acidosis decreases hemoglobin's affinity for oxygen, causing more release of oxygen contributing to sickling. Acidosis also causes less oxygen to be picked up by circulating hemoglobin in the lungs, further contributing to decreased pO_2.

   Increased osmolality causes sickling due to resultant cellular dehydration and increased HbS content within the cells. Increased osmolality also causes sluggish blood flow, contributing to hypoxemia, vascular obstruction, and further sickling.

   In reversible sickle cells, the membranes will return to normal when the pO_2 of the blood returns to normal. In irreversible sickle cells, the membranes stay in the elongated crescent shape because of calcium ion influx.

CHAPTER

22

Structure and Function of the Cardiovascular and Lymphatic Systems

OBJECTIVES

After review of this chapter, the learner will be able to:

1. **Diagram the circulatory system and state the functions of each circuit.**

2. **Describe the cardiac cycle.**

3. **Discuss the four unique characteristics of the myocardial cells and conduction system: automaticity, rhythmicity, conductivity, and contractility.**

4. **Use the Frank-Starling law and Laplace's law to demonstrate the interrelationship between preload, afterload, and contractility.**

5. **Describe the similarities and differences in structure and function of arteries, veins, and capillaries.**

6. **Describe the role of the endothelium for control of vessel contraction or relaxation.**

7. **Discuss the factors influencing the systemic blood pressure.**

8. **Discuss the normal structure and function of the lymphatic system.**

LECTURE OUTLINE	INSTRUCTOR'S NOTES

The Circulatory System
The Heart
    Structures that direct circulation through the heart
        The heart wall
        Chambers of the heart
        Fibrous skeleton of the heart
        Valves of the heart
        The great vessels
        Blood flow during the cardiac cycle
        Normal intracardiac pressures
    Structures that support cardiac metabolism:
        the coronary vessels
        Coronary arteries
        Collateral arteries
        Coronary capillaries
        Coronary veins and lymphatic vessels
    Structures that control heart action
        The conduction system
        Cardiac innervation
        Myocardial cells
        Myocardial contraction and relaxation
    Factors affecting cardiac performance

LECTURE OUTLINE	INSTRUCTOR'S NOTES

Frank-Starling law of the heart
 Laplace's law
 Preload
 Afterload
 Heart rate
 Myocardial contractility
 Factors determining cardiac output
The Systemic Circulation
 Structure of blood vessels
  Arterial vessels
  Control of vessel contraction of relaxation:
   vasomotion
  Veins
 Factors affecting blood flow
  Pressure and resistance
  Neural control of total peripheral resistance
  Velocity
  Laminar versus turbulent flow
  Vascular compliance
 Regulation of blood pressure
  Arterial pressure
  Venous pressure
 Regulation of the coronary circulation
  Autoregulation
  Autonomic regulation
The Lymphatic System

DIFFICULT CONCEPTS

Reinforcing the Use of Physical Laws as They Relate to Cardiac Function (e.g., Frank-Starling law of the heart, Laplace's law)

 Whenever possible, these physical laws should be reinforced for learning hemodynamics and alterations of hemodynamics. For example, using Laplace's law, or the law of Laplace, to show how an aneurysm develops provides the understanding of the hemodynamics involved. A picture of a cylinder identifying the radius (r), wall thickness (c), and tension (t) produced because of wall thickness and a picture of a distensible cylinder (to represent the heart or a blood vessel) with the wall not as thick and bulging (aneurysm formation) can help students see the radius become greater (where the bulge is), causing greater tension on the wall and, presumably, causing the formation of an aneurysm. Illustrating the normal laws in Chapter 21 with appropriate short, uncomplicated examples in Chapter 22 helps students understand and apply the information.

Autonomic Control of Cardiovascular Function

 Sometimes, the autonomic nervous system has not been reviewed adequately prior to the cardiovascular disorders. Prior to the pathophysiology, it is helpful if about an hour is spent reviewing normal autonomic function. Included in this discussion are the vasomotor function of the sympathetic nervous system, differences and similarities between alpha and beta receptors, sympathetic and parasympathetic activation of the heart and blood vessels, and autonomic regulation during emergency situations (e.g., low perfusion pressure). Students find this content difficult. For example, why, with adrenergic stimulation of the beta receptors in the conduction system of the heart, is the result an increase in heart rate? They think this can happen only if it's an alpha receptor. So, spending time on this area prior to discussing hypertension, heart failure, dysrhythmias, and shock helps demystify consequent clinical manifestations.

CRITICAL THINKING

1. Using the Frank-Starling Law of the Heart describe how heart failure occurs.

   Answer: The Frank-Starling Law of the Heart proposes the length-tension relationship of cardiac muscle. It states that sarcomere length at the end of diastole determines tension generation, force of contraction of the next systole. Factors that increase contractility cause the heart to operate at a higher length-tension curve. The relationship between stretch and contraction can be likened to a rubber band. The more it is stretched, the faster it will recoil—up to a point. Eventually the fibers in the rubber band, much like cardiac muscle fibers, become over-stretched. Recoil, or contraction, decreases. In cardiac muscle, excessive stretching causes actin and myosin fibers to become partially disengaged disrupting crossbridges. This decreases the force of contraction. Higher and higher filling pressures are needed to provide normal contractile force. This is the positive feedback loop of congestive heart failure.

Alterations of Cardiovascular Function

OBJECTIVES

After review of this chapter, the learner will be able to:

1. Compare the physiologic effects of hypotension and hypertension.

2. Describe the various alterations in vascular flow (including thrombi, emboli, traumatic injury, atherosclerotic plaques, vasospastic disease, and varicosities) with the identification of outcomes such as stasis ulcers, chronic insufficiencies, and superior vena cava syndrome.

3. Identify the risk factors for atherosclerosis.

4. Discuss the progression of atherosclerotic heart disease from risk factor identification through the complications of acute myocardial infarction.

5. Describe dilated, hypertrophic, and restrictive cardiomyopathy.

6. Describe how a person contracts acute rheumatic fever and how it leads to rheumatic heart disease.

7. Compare right and left heart failure, including causation, manifestations, treatment, and complications.

8. Define dysrhythmia and state its significance.

9. Identify and describe the different types of shock.

10. Describe the progression from sepsis through septic shock to multisystem organ dysfunction syndrome.

LECTURE OUTLINE	INSTRUCTOR'S NOTES

Diseases of the Arteries and Veins
    Arteriosclerosis
    Atherosclerosis
    Hypertension
        Factors associated with primary hypertension
    Orthostatic (postural) hypotension
    Aneurysm
    Thrombus formation
    Embolism
    Peripheral arterial disease
        Thromboangiitis obliterans (Buerger disease)
        Raynaud phenomenon and disease
    Diseases of the veins
        Varicose veins and chronic venous
            insufficiency
        Thrombus formation in veins
        Superior vena cava syndrome

Coronary artery disease, myocardial ischemia, and
    myocardial infarction
    Development of coronary artery disease
    Myocardial ischemia
    Myocardial infarction
Disorders of the Heart Wall
    Disorders of the pericardium
        Acute pericarditis
        Pericardial effusion
        Constrictive pericarditis
    Disorders of the myocardium: the cardiomyopathies
    Disorders of the endocardium
        Valvular dysfunction
        Acute rheumatic fever and rheumatic heart
          disease
        Infective endocarditis
    Cardiac complications in acquired immuno-
        deficiency syndrome (AIDS)
Manifestations of Heart Disease
    Dysrhythmias
    Heart failure
        Types
Shock
    Impairment of Cellular Metabolism
        Impairment of oxygen use
        Impairment of glucose use
    Types of shock and multiple dysfunction syndrome
        Cardiogenic shock
        Hypovolemic shock
        Neurogenic shock
        Anaphylactic shock
        Septic shock
    Treatment for shock
    Multiple organ dysfunction syndrome

DIFFICULT CONCEPTS

Hypertension

A thorough way to help students understand the major factors responsible for increasing or decreasing blood pressure is to discuss the following equation, that is, Poiseuille's formula:

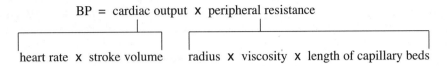

$$BP = \text{cardiac output} \times \text{peripheral resistance}$$

heart rate × stroke volume   radius × viscosity × length of capillary beds

Discuss each of these factors (except length of capillary beds; discuss this as a constant, since we really don't know how it changes and affects blood pressure) singularly and in combination with other factors (e.g., heart rate x stroke volume). With the equation, use examples; this helps students understand and not just memorize how certain conditions cause or result in high or low blood pressure. With this equation, students readily understand what kind of problems are fundamentally cardiac output problems or peripheral resistance problems, or both.

Heart Failure and Regression to Shock

Helpful for teaching heart failure is reinforcing the application of the Frank-Starling Law. Showing a slide or diagram of changes in the volume tension relationships as the heart fails and, for example, left ventricular preload increases causing disengagement of the contractile proteins helps students understand the involved hemodynamics. Perhaps the most difficult kind of shock to understand is septic shock. Figure 23-47 can help outline the progression of septic shock; however, students may need to review aspects of inflammation (e.g., functions of specific cytokines).

Multiple Organ Dysfunction Syndrome (MODS)

Much new information is now available about the pathogenesis of MODS. Once again, most problematic for new learners is mastery of immune/inflammatory content. Figure 23-48 outlines the pathogenesis of MODS. The same outline given to students in class helps them follow the progression.

CRITICAL THINKING

1. Explain the progressive pathophysiologic relationship between a myocardial infarction and the development of left ventricular (LV) failure. What factors affect the severity of LV failure?

Answer: A myocardial infarction (MI) is caused by irreversible hypoxia that leads to cellular death and necrosis. The zone of necrosis is immediately surrounded by a zone of hypoxic injury and an outer zone of ischemia. The necrotic area is comprised of dead tissue with damaged cell membranes. Enzymes leak from the damaged membranes into the lymph and subsequently into the blood. The process of inflammation begins immediately after the event with the infiltration of neutrophils. The destroyed cells in the zone of necrosis are degraded and replaced with scar tissue. In the zone of necrosis, the myofibrils no longer function, leading to an area of hypokinesis in the myocardial wall. In the zone of hypoxic injury and zone of ischemia, the injured myofibrils are oxygen deprived. Although not irreversibly damaged, they are unable to function normally. This leads to an area that either is unable to contract or contracts in a dysfunctional manner.

In summary, the damage to the myocardial muscle causes decreased cardiac contractility in the area of the infarction, decreased LV compliance, decreased LV stroke volume, increased LV preload (LV end-diastolic pressure), and myocardial conduction abnormalities. The degree of dysfunction is dependent on the size and site of the MI as well as the presence or absence of any other myocardial scar tissue.

An MI contributes to the development of LV failure because of the damage to the left ventricle. The decreased contractility as a result of the infarction causes the blood pressure and volume in the left ventricle to rise. This rise in volume and pressure causes blood to "back up," increasing preload. As a result, left atrial volume and pressure rise. The blood coming from the coronary veins into the left atrium meets rising pressure. Again this causes a "back up" with increased volume and pressure in the pulmonary capillary bed. The high fluid pressure (hydrostatic pressure) in the pulmonary capillaries causes water to move into the interstitium and alveoli. This decreases oxygen-carbon dioxide diffusion which decreases pO_2 and causes the myocardial muscle to become more hypoxic, further perpetuating the cycle. As the pressure rises in the lungs, the "back up" affects the right ventricle, right atrium, and systemic venous system respectively.

The decreased stroke volume and decreased ejection fraction of the left ventricle also cause a decrease in cardiac output. In order to maintain blood pressure, systemic vascular resistance will increase by catecholamine release and sodium and water retention. Catecholamines (epinephrine and norepinephrine) increase systemic vascular resistance via arterial vasoconstriction. They also increase myocardial ischemia because of increased cardiac work related to resultant tachycardia. At the same time, the juxtaglomerular apparatus of the kidney releases renin, an enzyme which converts angiotensinogen to angiotensin. Angiotensin is a potent vasoconstrictor and stimulates the release of aldosterone which retains sodium and water. The rising systemic vascular resistance increases afterload, and the increased work of the left ventricle causes further ischemia.

Over time, this cycle of failure and increasing ischemia will tax the body's ability to compensate and systemic blood pressure will fall. This further decreases oxygenation and increases hypoxia.

2. Explain how cellular metabolism is impaired in sepsis syndrome.

Answer: In sepsis syndrome, cellular metabolism is impaired by the response of target cells to the chemicals of inflammation, the presence of multiple mediators of inflammation, and the ability of the target cell to release these mediators of inflammation. Infective agents, either bacterial or viral, directly and indirectly injure cells. Cells directly invaded by the agent may be damaged and unable to function normally. If the agent is bacterial, endotoxins are released into the bloodstream, interrupting cellular metabolism, causing cellular damage, and releasing cellular enzymes and lysosomes.

Implicated in the genesis of septic shock are several chemicals: interleukins, tumor necrosis factor, platelet-activating factor, and myocardial depressant substance. These chemicals initiate a process of increased capillary permeability and vasodilation. In sepsis syndrome, vasodilation is massive, with peripheral pooling and decreased systemic vascular resistance (SVR). This causes decreased blood return to the heart, peripheral stagnation, and tissue hypoxemia. The lowered SVR also decreases afterload.

Although endotoxin from the infectious agent can directly cause the hypothalamus to induce fever and produce the characteristic vasodilation, the generation of shock from bacteremia is dependent on several of the above-mentioned chemicals. The fever increases tissue basal metabolic rate and increases tissue oxygen demand. The combination of the decreased afterload, increased tissue oxygen demand, and decreased blood pressure causes the heart to increase its work in order to compensate. In sepsis syndrome, cardiac output markedly increases, causing increased myocardial work until myocardial depressant factor impairs myocardial contractility. Despite the myocardial work, the hypoxemia is profound, leading to anaerobic cellular metabolism and increasing lactic acidosis.

Alterations of Cardiovascular Function in Children

OBJECTIVES

After review of this chapter, the learner will be able to:

1. **Identify the risk factors for congenital cardiac defects.**

2. **Describe cyanotic and acyanotic congenital heart defects.**

3. **Differentiate between congenital heart defects that increase, decrease, or do not change pulmonary blood flow.**

4. **Discuss rheumatic heart disease in childhood.**

LECTURE OUTLINE	INSTRUCTOR'S NOTES

Congenital Heart Diseases
    Obstructive defects
        Coarctation of the aorta
        Aortic stenosis
        Pulmonic stenosis
    Defects with increased pulmonary blood flow
        Patent ductus arteriosus
        Atrial septal defect
        Ventricular septal defect
        Atrioventricular canal defect
    Mixed Defects
        Transposition of the great arteries or
            transposition of the great vessels
        Total anomalous pulmonary venous
            connection
        Truncus arteriosus
        Hypoplastic left heart syndrome
    Defects with decreased pulmonary blood flow
        Tetralogy of Fallot
        Tricuspid atresia
    Congestive heart failure
Acquired Cardiovascular Disorders
    Kawasaki disease
    Systemic hypertension

DIFFICULT CONCEPTS

Hemodynamics of the Congenital Heart Defects

Without a doubt this content is always confusing. Using the figures of hemodynamic changes (giving students an illustration of each type of congenital heart defect), trace the flow of blood identifying the altered pressures and volumes. Sometimes giving students a blank copy (i.e., without the altered pressures) of the schematics used in Figure 23-3 for each defect and asking them to determine subsequent flow, pressure alterations, etc., reinforces their understanding of the relationships among pressure, flow, and resistance.

Hypertension in Children

A preamble explaining how little is really known about childhood blood pressure is often useful to this content. For example, the initial graphs assessing blood pressure in children was plotted against age. Over time with new research (the Bogalusa studies), higher accuracy was achieved for assessing blood pressure with the variables of height and weight. Thus, it was the children with increased body mass who revealed higher-than- normal blood pressures. Stressing the correlation of inactivity and poor diet to high blood pressure in children and how these variables, often overlooked in children, contribute to hypertension in the adult is important. How different mechanisms of action vary with race should also be emphasized.

CRITICAL THINKING

1. A neonate has a harsh, loud, systolic murmur shortly after birth. It is best heard at the left lower sternal border. The neonate is acyanotic and has no other symptoms. What type of congenital heart disorder does this infant have? Explain why the neonate is not cyanotic. When could the infant become cyanotic?

   Answer: The neonate has a ventricular septal defect (VSD). It is an acyanotic congenital heart defect occurring in the interventricular septum. Because the pressure in the left ventricle is greater than in the right ventricle, the blood will flow from left/oxygenated to right/unoxygenated. Therefore, the blood leaving the left ventricle through the aorta is oxygenated blood, so the infant will be acyanotic. The left-to-right shunt causes mixed oxygenated and unoxygenated blood to flow into the lungs. This increased flow leads to increasing pulmonary vascular resistance and pulmonary hypertension.

   Cyanosis occurs when the infant develops congestive heart failure with subsequent hypoxemia. Cyanosis may also occur if the VSD is large. With a large VSD, the pressures in the left and right ventricles can equalize. The shunt will be determined by which side of the heart has the greatest resistance. If the right ventricle has higher pulmonary resistance, the shunt will be right-to-left, causing cyanosis because blood is shunted to the left ventricle instead of to the lungs.

2. Why do children with Tetralogy of Fallot have cyanosis? Why do they squat? Explain the pathophysiology and anatomic features involved.

   Answer: Tetralogy of Fallot is a cyanotic heart defect with four anatomic abnormalities: a large VSD, an overriding aorta, pulmonary stenosis, and right ventricular hypertrophy. Blood flows into the right ventricle, but the pulmonary stenosis causes an outflow obstruction and prevents adequate amounts of blood to flow into the pulmonary artery. Therefore, a right-to-left shunt is created, causing unoxygenated blood from the right ventricle to flow unimpeded into the aorta through the VSD. Also, the amount of oxygenated blood coming into the left ventricle from the lungs is decreased. Shunt direction varies according to changes in pressure and the size of the various defects. If systemic pressure exceeds the pressure of the stenotic pulmonary artery, the shunt will reverse.

   Squatting is a compensatory mechanism used by children to stop hypoxic or "tet" spells. By squatting, children increase their systemic vascular resistance (SVR). The increased SVR changes the shunt in the ventricular septal defect (VSD) to a left-to-right shunt. The increased SVR also decreases blood return to the heart through the inferior vena cava. This mechanism will temporarily decrease cyanosis.

CHAPTER

25

Structure and Function of the Pulmonary System

OBJECTIVES

After review of this chapter, the learner will be able to:

1. Identify the structures that participate in gas exchange and are collectively called the acinus.

2. Describe the protective structures that surround the pulmonary system.

3. Identify the factors essential to successful ventilation, perfusion, and diffusion.

4. Discuss the properties of compliance and elastic recoil as they relate to the normal function of the lung in ventilation.

5. Describe the neurochemical regulation of ventilation.

6. Describe the mechanics of breathing.

7. Discuss the importance of the oxyhemoglobin dissociation curve for evaluating effective gas exchange.

8. Describe the movement and transport forms of carbon dioxide from the body tissues to the lungs.

9. Discuss ventilation/perfusion mechanisms.

10. Identify the determinants of arterial oxygenation.

LECTURE OUTLINE	INSTRUCTOR'S NOTES

Structures of the Pulmonary System
    Conducting airways
    Gas-exchange airways
    Pulmonary and bronchial circulation
    Chest wall and pleura
Function of the Pulmonary System
    Ventilation
        Measurement of gas pressure
        Lung volumes and capacities
    Neurochemical control of ventilation
        Lung receptors
        Chemoreceptors
        Mechanics of breathing
            Major and accessory muscles
            Alveolar surface tension
            Elastic properties of the lung and chest
                wall
            Airway resistance
            Work of breathing
    Gas transport
        Distribution of ventilation and perfusion

<table>
<tr><td>**LECTURE OUTLINE**</td><td>**INSTRUCTOR'S NOTES**</td></tr>
</table>

DIFFICULT CONCEPTS

The Trachea

The structure of the airways can be viewed as an inverted tree. Two major branches represent the trachea with further branching for the major bronchi and the many subdivisions of the bronchi leading to the alveoli. A bunch of grapes can represent the alveolar ducts, alveolar sacs, and alveoli. The stem represents the alveolar ducts; each cluster of grapes represents an alveolar sac; and each grape represents an alveolus.

Ventilation and Perfusion Relationships

Changes in the relationship between ventilation and pulmonary blood flow (perfusion) can be difficult for students to understand, particularly concepts of dead space effect and shunt effect in the lung. Dead space effect is the result of inadequate blood flowing through the lungs with decreased amounts of blood to exchange with air. The result of ventilation in excess of perfusion is like trucks of wheat being delivered to the railroad station (ventilation) where railroad cars (red blood cell perfusion) haul the wheat away for utilization by the greater population (the body). If there are not enough railroad cars for the amount of wheat delivered to the depot, there will be a decrease in the amount of wheat transported to the railroad cars and a decrease in the amount of wheat available to the greater population. The problem of shunt effect can be likened to the wheat not being able to get to the railroad station because the road is obstructed in some way. The railroad cars are sent to another delivery point (shunted) where the roads are open and the wheat can be transferred.

Ventilation, Diffusion, and Perfusion

Understanding the relationships among structures of the bronchial tree, the alveoli, and the pulmonary capillary system is necessary if students are to understand how these relationships are altered with disease states. When describing the relationship between ventilation perfusion and diffusion, the use of Figure 24-6 is helpful. The relationship between the alveolar structure and the pulmonary capillary assists students to understand how ventilation and perfusion are functionally related and the factors that affect diffusion. Students can better appreciate concepts related to pulmonary edema, pulmonary embolism, and atelectasis when they understand the significance of the structural relationships at the alveolar capillary membrane.

Compliance and Work of Breathing

The relationship between changes in compliance and work of breathing is often confusing to students. The example of new and used balloons is often helpful. A small, new balloon is difficult to inflate with air (decreased compliance). It requires a lot of respiratory effort or air pressure to blow up the balloon. This is like a lung unit with low compliance, or a stiff lung. It helps students to understand that balloons with a small radius require more air pressure to inflate. Comparatively, after the balloon has been blown up several times, the elastic of the balloon becomes overstretched and the balloon is flabby and retains air (increased compliance). It takes relatively less respiratory work to blow up the balloon, but when you let go of the balloon it does not sail around the room with the force of expiring air as a new balloon does; and when it finally hits the floor, there is air remaining in the balloon. Therefore, it is like high compliance in the lung with loss of elasticity and air trapping. The effort, or work, of breathing for high compliance is in getting air out of the lung. Being able to see the air remaining in the flabby balloon helps students understand the concept of air trapping in obstructive disease (increased work of expiration). With the new, small balloon, the effort is in inflating the balloon (increased work of inspiration).

CO_2 narcosis and the danger of administering oxygen are sometimes confusing concepts. The loss of sensitivity of the CO_2 receptors can be likened to the loss of sensitivity or awareness of the elastic in your underwear. Students won't be aware that they have their underwear on because the sensory receptors become fatigued from the constant pressure; likewise the CO_2 receptors will become fatigued with constantly high levels of CO_2 and will no longer provide a protective stimulus for ventilation.

CRITICAL THINKING

1. Explain the changes that occur in the pulmonary system with aging.

   Answer: Chest wall compliance decreases because the ribs become ossified and joints grow stiffer. Kyphoscoliosis may curve the vertebral column changing the shape of the thoracic cage. Elastic recoil of the lungs diminishes. This results is increased lung compliance and reduced ventilation capacity, increased residual volumes, reduced ventilatory reserves, and decreased ventilation-perfusion ratios. But, total lung capacity is unchanged.

   Maximum PaO2 decreases to 0.3 times age minus 100 (at sea level). Pulmonary capillary networks decrease. There is decreased surface area for gas exchange.

   Decreased PaO2 and ventilatory reserve lead to decreased exercise tolerance. Early airway closure inhibits expiratory flow. Changes depend on activity and fitness levels in earlier life. Decreased respiratory muscle strength and endurance can still be enhanced by exercise.

CHAPTER

26

Alterations of Pulmonary Function

OBJECTIVES

After review of this chapter, the learner will be able to:

1. Define hyper- and hypoventilation.

2. Describe atelectasis and give two specific causes.

3. Describe the pleural abnormalities of pneumathorax, pleural effusion, empyema, and pleurisy.

4. List conditions outside of the pulmonary system that directly affect pulmonary function.

5. Differentiate between hypoxia and hypoxemia.

6. Describe adult respiratory distress syndrome.

7. Describe common consequences of the obstructive pulmonary diseases.

8. Discuss the similarities and differences between the pneumonias and tuberculosis.

9. Describe the cellular changes, clinical manifestations, treatments, outcomes, and complications of pulmonary embolus.

10. Describe the different types of lung cancer.

LECTURE OUTLINE	INSTRUCTOR'S NOTES

Clinical Manifestations of Pulmonary Alterations
   Signs and symptoms of pulmonary disease
      Dyspnea
      Abnormal breathing patterns
      Hypoventilation/hyperventilation
      Cough
      Hemoptysis
      Cyanosis
      Pain
      Clubbing
      Abnormal sputum
   Conditions caused by pulmonary disease or injury
      Hypercapnia
      Hypoxemia
      Acute respiratory failure
      Pulmonary edema
      Aspiration
      Atelectasis
      Brochiectasis
      Bronchiolitis
      Pleural abnormalities
      Abscess formation and cavitation

LECTURE OUTLINE	INSTRUCTOR'S NOTES

Pulmonary fibrosis
Chest wall restriction
Flail chest
Inhalation disorders
Pulmonary Disorders
    Acute respiratory failure
        Acute respiratory distress syndrome
        Postoperative respiratory failure
    Obstructive pulmonary disease
        Asthma
        Chronic bronchitis
        Emphysema
    Respiratory tract infections
        Pneumonia
        Tuberculosis
        Acute bronchitis
    Pulmonary vascular disease
        Pulmonary embolism
        Pulmonary hypertension
        Cor pulmonale
    Lip cancer
    Laryngeal cancer
    Lung cancer
        Types of lung cancer
        Staging of lung cancer

DIFFICULT CONCEPTS

Upper and Lower Airway Obstruction

Differences in the causes of inspiratory and expiratory obstruction and upper and lower airway disorders may be puzzling to students. A barbell-shaped balloon with one of the barbells in a vacuum bottle can serve as an illustration of the relationship between changes in intrathoracic pressure and environmental air pressure that contributes to collapse of airways and symptoms of wheezing or stridor. The creation of a vacuum in a bottle (intrathoracic negative pressure) causes the balloon and the neck of the balloon to expand within the bottle. Simultaneously, the vacuum is transferred to the balloon outside the bottle causing it to collapse, which is analogous to air in the upper air passages outside the thorax. This illustrates how the negative pressure of a vacuum (inspiration) is transmitted to the air passage of the balloon outside the bottle (outside the thorax) causing it to collapse (inspiratory stridor). However, when the vacuum in the bottle is released and air is forced out of the balloon in the vacuum bottle, the airway to the balloon outside of the bottle opens. The neck of the balloon in the bottle tends to collapse (expiratory wheezing) as a result of the positive pressures around the airways, ultimately causing obstruction to airflow before all of the air can get out (air trapping).

Obstruction and Air Trapping

Concepts of obstruction and air trapping are basic to the pathophysiologic mechanisms underlying asthma, chronic obstructive bronchitis, emphysema, and tension pneumothorax. A ball valve analogy can be useful for explaining collapse of airways that occurs with the change from negative to positive intrathoracic pressure with expiration. The widening of the airways that occurs with inspiration, or the opening in the pleura with a pneumothorax, is analogous to the air intake through a pipe with a ball valve. With expiration the ball valve closes, which results in obstruction with accumulation of air behind the ball, similar to narrowing of airways on expiration or the closure of the pleural opening of a pneumothorax as intrathoracic pressure changes from negative to positive.

CRITICAL THINKING

1. Analyze the similarities and differences between emphysema and chronic bronchitis.

   Answer: Both chronic bronchitis and emphysema can be caused by irritants such as cigarette smoke or other air pollutants. They are characterized by air trapping and obstruction that lead to hypoxemia, hypoventilation, and abnormal ventilation-perfusion ratio. They can lead to congestive heart failure. Their symptoms include dyspnea, decreased exercise tolerance, frequent infections, and fatigue.

   Chronic bronchitis is characterized by increased mucus production, mucosal edema, impaired or lost ciliary function, and a chronic cough lasting at least 3 months per year for 2 years. The inspired irritants cause a chronic inflammatory response and mucosal edema. The inflammation and irritants increase the size and number of mucus and goblet cells in the epithelial cells of the airways, producing thicker, more viscous, and larger amounts of mucus. The thick mucus then impairs ciliary function.

   Emphysema is caused by elastin breakdown that destroys lung tissue, occurring in the alveolar septa or respiratory bronchioles. This process destroys alveolar and respiratory bronchiole integrity and obliterates pulmonary capillaries. The loss of elastic recoil inherent in lung tissue, hyperinflation of the alveoli, and decreased diameter of the bronchioles leads to air trapping.

2. Mr. Rusch is being evaluated for multiple pulmonary emboli. What risk factors and clinical findings are commonly associated with pulmonary emboli?

   Answer: The major risk factors for the development of pulmonary emboli are venous stasis, hypercoagulability states, and bleeding injuries or lesions. Examples of venous stasis factors include immobility, pregnancy, congestive heart failure, obesity, sickle cell anemia, and systemic lupus erythematosus. Examples of hypercoagulability states include polycythemia vera, dehydration, coagulation disorders, and oral contraceptive use. Examples of bleeding injuries or lesions include strokes, surgery, and traumatic injuries. Lower extremity thrombophlebitis is commonly associated with and a predisposing factor for pulmonary emboli. The symptoms associated with lower extremity thrombophlebitis include edema, red or dusky coloration, calf pain on palpation, and positive Homan's sign.

   The clinical findings associated with pulmonary emboli include dyspnea, tachypnea, tachycardia, unexplained anxiety, and pleural pain. If there is lung infarction, symptoms will also include fever, pleural friction rub, pleural effusion, hemoptysis, and leukocytosis. Massive pulmonary emboli will cause hypotension, chest pain, and profound shock.

Alterations of Pulmonary Function in Children

OBJECTIVES

After review of this chapter, the learner will be able to:

1. Describe the significant differences between the pulmonary systems of infants and children and that found in a normal adult.

2. Compare the two major types of croup, laryngotracheobronchitis, and epiglottitis, with reference to the differential diagnosis, treatment, and prognosis.

3. Identify how the allergic response can trigger childhood asthma attacks.

4. Describe bronchiolitis obliterans.

5. Discuss the causes of bronchopulmonary dysplasia in the premature neonate.

6. Describe the pathophysiology, clinical manifestations, and treatment for a child with cystic fibrosis.

7. Describe sudden infant death syndrome.

LECTURE OUTLINE	INSTRUCTOR'S NOTES

Pulmoanry Disorders
    Disorders of the Upper Airways
        Infections (Croup syndromes)
        Aspiration of foreign bodies
        Aspiration of foreign substances
    Disorders of the lower airways
        Respiratory distress syndrome
        Asthma
        Respiratory infections
        Bronchopulmonary dysplasia
        Cystic fibrosis
    Sudden infant death syndrome (SIDS)

DIFFICULT CONCEPTS

Croup Syndromes and Airway Obstruction

Croup syndromes are the most common cause of airway obstruction in young children. Students understand that respiratory stridor will first occur on inspiration when they have clarification that airways outside the thorax tend to collapse from negative pressure that is transferred from the thorax during inspiration. This can be illustrated by sucking air through a 6-inch length of 1/2-inch penrose drain tubing and a 6-inch length of 5/8-inch bore garden hose. The penrose drain tubing will collapse because the softness of the structure cannot resist the negative air pressure. The length of garden hose will remain open. The penrose drain tubing is like the less mature soft cartilage and smaller lumen of a young child's inflamed upper airway, while the garden hose is more like the larger lumen and firm cartilage of adult upper airways.

Asthma and Airway Obstruction

Students can be assisted to understand the airway obstruction of asthma by reviewing the process of the inflammatory response occurring in the smaller airways. Integrating what they have learned about inflammation in Chapter 6 helps to apply general concepts to specific pathophysiologic conditions.

Lack of Surfactant and Respiratory Distress Syndrome

Lack of surfactant and decreased surface tension are important and difficult concepts related to collapse of airways in infant respiratory distress syndrome. The concept of how surfactant decreases surface tension can be demonstrated by placing a drop of liquid detergent in water that is covered by a thin film of cooking oil. The soap will cause the film of oil to disperse. Soap bubbles can also be used to illustrate how surfactant reduces the force of attraction between water molecules and, thus, helps prevent collapse of alveoli during ventilation.

CRITICAL THINKING

1. A 2-year-old child is diagnosed with cystic fibrosis. How would alterations in her exocrine glands influence her breathing?

   Answer: Cystic fibrosis is an autosomal recessive disease of the exocrine glands causing the excessive production of thick mucus. In the child's lungs, the thick mucus causes bronchiolar obstruction, mucus plugging, and atelectasis. Her airway walls are destroyed with air trapping. She is predisposed to frequent infections and develops chronic inflammation. This leads to increased dyspnea, frequent chronic cough, and sputum production.

2. Explain why croup is primarily a disease of children.

   Answer: Croup is a clinical syndrome manifested by an infection of the upper airways. Children are more apt to have croup because they have a more immature immune system. Their airways and glottis are small in diameter. The mucous membrane lining their upper airways is more loosely attached and vascular. Their cartilaginous rings collapse more easily. With edema and inflammation, they are easily compromised. The general surface area of children's lungs is less, which limits their pulmonary compensation. Because their submucosa contains many lymphoid cells, children are more apt to develop edema and swelling if inflammation occurs.

CHAPTER

28

Structure and Function of the Renal and Urologic Systems

OBJECTIVES

After review of this chapter, the learner will be able to:

1. Describe the anatomy of the renal system.

2. Diagram the structures and major functions of the nephron.

3. Describe the mechanisms regulating glomerular filtration rate.

4. List the four processes integral to urine formation.

5. Identify the electrolytes reabsorbed and secreted by the proximal and distal tubes.

6. Describe the countercurrent exchange system of urine concentration.

7. Identify hormones activated or secreted by the kidney and describe their actions.

8. Discuss the clinical significance of blood urea nitrogen and creatinine measurements.

LECTURE OUTLINE	INSTRUCTOR'S NOTES

Structures of the Renal System
    Structures of the kidney
        Nephron
        Blood vessels of the kidney
    Urinary structures
        Ureters
        Bladder and urethra
Renal Blood Flow
    Autoregulation
    Neural regulation
    Hormonal regulation
Kidney Function
    Nephron function
        Glomerular filtration
    Concentration and dilution of urine
        Water, sodium, and chloride
        Urea
        Urine
        Antidiuretic hormone (ADH)
        Diuretics as a factor in urine flow
    Renal hormones
        Vitamin D
        Erythropoietin
        Atrial natriuretic hormone

LECTURE OUTLINE	INSTRUCTOR'S NOTES

The concept of clearance
    Clearance and glomerular filtration rate
    Plasma creatinine concentration
    Blood urea nitrogen

DIFFICULT CONCEPTS

The Functions of the Kidney

The analogy of a combined water treatment and garbage disposal facility linked to an efficient recycling center can help students comprehend the "big picture" of kidney function and the urinary drainage system in regulating the internal environment of the body. Most chemical exchanges with the blood occur in the kidneys, where they filter, secrete, reabsorb, and excrete chemicals and water to produce urine. The waste stream entering the garbage disposal/recycling plant is carefully screened, with some materials totally discarded and some retained on a limited basis. Extensive effort is expended to recapture valuable substances. This analogy can be used to explain both normal urinary function and many pathological responses seen in disease states. In effect, the kidneys serve to launder the body fluids of liquid sewage and, at the same time, retain essential chemicals and nutrients. It is sometimes said that the composition of body fluids is determined not so much by what we eat and drink as by what the kidneys keep or excrete.

Glomerular Capillaries-Bowman's Capsule Relationships

Making a fist of your fingers to form a knot of "glomerular capillaries" and pushing it into an inflated balloon simulates a glomerulus. The inner surface of Bowman's capsule is pressed against your fingers and the air in the balloon represents Bowman's space. The outer surface of the balloon forms the outer wall of Bowman's capsule, which in the actual nephron is continuous with the wall of the proximal convoluted tubule.

CRITICAL THINKING

1. Explain the countercurrent exchange system of concentrating and diluting urine.

Answer: In countercurrent exchange fluid flows in opposite directions in parallel tubes. In the thick ascending loop of Henle sodium and chloride move out by active transport into the medullary interstitium. As the hypoosmotic fluid moves into the descending tubule the hyperosmotic medullary interstitium pulls water from the tubule. The efficiency of water conservation is related to the lengths of the loops. The longer the loops, the greater the ability to concentrate urine.

Alterations of Renal and Urinary Tract Function

OBJECTIVES

After review of this chapter, the learner will be able to:

1. Discuss the causes and effects of obstructions in various locations within the urinary tract.

2. Describe the two most common tumors of the renal and urologic systems: renal carcinoma and bladder tumors.

3. Discuss the etiology, infectious agents, manifestations, treatments, and complications of urinary tract infections.

4. Describe acute and chronic pyelonephritis.

5. Identify the causes of glomerulonephritis and the resulting changes in glomerular structure and function.

6. Discuss the similarities and differences between acute, rapidly progressive, and chronic glomerulonephritis.

7. Describe nephrotic syndrome from causation through complications.

8. Differentiate between prerenal, intrarenal, and postrenal causes of acute renal failure.

9. Discuss the clinical manifestations, treatment options, outcomes, and complications of acute renal failure.

10. Discuss the multiple system manifestations of chronic renal failure.

LECTURE OUTLINE	INSTRUCTOR'S NOTES

Urinary Tract Obstruction
    Consequences of obstruction
    Obstructive disorders
        Kidney stones
        Neurogenic bladder
    Tumors
        Renal tumors
        Bladder tumors
Urinary Tract Infection
    Causes of urinary tract infection
    Types of urinary tract infection
        Cystitis
        "Nonbacterial" cystitis
        Acute pyelonephritis
        Chronic pyelonephritis
Glomerular Disorders
    Glomerulonephritis
        Types of glomerulonephritis
    Nephrotic syndrome

LECTURE OUTLINE	INSTRUCTOR'S NOTES

Renal Failure
    Classification of renal dysfunction
    Types of renal failure
        Acute renal failure
        Chronic renal failure

DIFFICULT CONCEPTS

Oliguria, Proteinuria, and Glomerulonephritis

Students studying glomerulonephritis frequently have difficulty understanding how there can be decreased glomerulofiltration rate with decreased urine formation concurrent with proteinuria and/or hematuria. An analogy of a rusty pipe can be helpful to them. A decrease of water flow through the pipe caused by the accumulation of deposits on the inside of the pipe is like decreased flow of blood through the glomerular capillaries as a consequence of tissue swelling from inflammation or accumulation of cells in the Bowman's space, which surround the capillaries, compressing them and also causing decreased flow. The rust can also cause perforations in the pipe, resulting in a leaky pipe. The leaky pipe is like the increased permeability of the glomerulocapillary membrane that allows proteins and/or red blood cells to pass through into the urine.

CRITICAL THINKING

1. Ms. Cornwall is admitted with pyelonephritis. She has chills and her temperature is 101° F. She is complaining of flank pain, frequency, and dysuria. Her urine has white blood cell casts and her urine culture is growing E. coli. Why does she have bacteria and white blood cell casts in her urine?

   Answer: Ms. Cornwall has a focal bacterial infection of her renal pelvis, calyces, and medulla. The bacterial invasion triggers an inflammatory reaction with white blood cell response causing edema and release of inflammatory mediators. In severe pyelonephritis, abscess formation and necrosis may occur in the medulla. Scar tissue may form with healing. The urine coming from the glomeruli mixes with inflammatory exudate in the renal pelvis and calyces or tubules with extensive infection. This leads to purulent urine with bacteria and white blood cell casts present.

2. What is the difference between prerenal acute renal failure, intrarenal acute renal failure, and postrenal acute renal failure? Give examples of each.

   Answer: Prerenal acute renal failure is decreased renal function with elevated blood urea nitrogen (BUN) and plasma creatinine due to impaired blood flow to the kidney. Blood flow and pressure reaching the afferent arteriole of the kidney are low, which causes a low glomerular filtration rate and eventual renal ischemia. Examples of prerenal acute renal failure causes include hypovolemia, hypotension, shock, hemorrhage, myocardial infarction with poor cardiac output, and left ventricular failure.

   Postrenal acute renal failure is caused by impaired outflow from the kidney. Urine's passage is blocked by an obstruction, causing urine to "back up" into the renal pelvis and changing pressures within the kidney. Examples are kidney stones, bladder outlet obstruction, and enlarged prostate.

   Intrarenal acute renal failure is caused by impaired blood flow within the kidney. It is the result of direct damage to the kidney, including ischemia or inflammatory damage. Examples of intrarenal causes include acute tubular necrosis (ATN), glomerulonephritis, malignant hypertension, disseminated intravascular coagulation (DIC), and renal vasculitis.

Alterations of Renal and Urinary Tract Function in Children

OBJECTIVES

After review of this chapter, the learner will be able to:

1. Describe the common congenital anomalies that occur within the renal and urologic systems.

2. Describe the manifestations of nephrotic syndrome, glomerulonephritis, and hemolytic uremic syndrome in children.

3. Describe the structural alterations that result in vesicoureteral reflex.

4. Describe Wilms' tumor.

5. Discuss the occurrence, patterns, and probable etiologies of enuresis.

LECTURE OUTLINE

INSTRUCTOR'S NOTES

Structural Abnormalities
    Hypospadias
    Epispadias with exstrophy of the bladder
    Hypoplastic/dysplastic kidneys
    Renal agenesis
Glomerular Disorders
    Nephrotic syndrome
    Glomerulonephritis
        Post streptococcal glomerulonephritis
        IgA nephropathy
    Hemolytic uremic syndrome
Obstructive Disorders
    Urinary tract infections
    Vesicoureteral reflux
Wilms' Tumor
Enuresis
    Types of enuresis

DIFFICULT CONCEPTS

Nephrotic Syndrome

Nephrotic syndrome is a classic example of how changes in plasma oncotic pressure influence the distribution of water among body compartments. Water can be retained with the formation of severe edema, but the water is not available for other body function.

Obstructive Disorders

Obstruction of urine flow may be caused by congenital malformations, inflammatory processes, or tumors. Regardless of the cause, there will be accumulation of urine behind the obstruction, leading to distention of the luminal structures and an alteration in the function of the surrounding structures. Students can enhance their critical thinking skills by tracing a drop of urine from the glomerulus to the external urethra and then discussing the consequences of an obstruction at any point along the path of urine flow.

CRITICAL THINKING

1. A 3-year-old child is admitted with primary nephrotic syndrome. What signs and symptoms would be identified? What is the primary treatment for this syndrome and why?

   Answer: The child would be lethargic, fatigued, and irritable. He would have generalized edema at night and dependent edema with protuberant abdomen during the day. The edema would eventually progress to excessive generalized edema with pulmonary congestion and genital swelling. He would have a decreased amount of frothy or foamy urine, diarrhea, anorexia, and malnutrition. His skin would be shiny and pale with hair changes. His blood pressure would be either normal or high. He would be more susceptible to infection. The primary treatment for nephrotic syndrome is the use of glucocorticoids (steroids) to decrease the inflammatory response.

2. While bathing a child, the parent discovers a firm, smooth mass on the child's flank. When touched, the mass is nontender. Otherwise, the child appears healthy and well. What type of mass does this child have and why?

   Answer: The child has Wilms' tumor, an embryonal tumor of the kidney. It arises from undifferentiated embryonic renal tubule and glomerular cells called metanephric blastemal cells. The error in development occurs between weeks 8 and 34 in the fetus. However, the tumor does not grow until after birth. With Wilms' tumor, the embryo-like cells grow in a rapid, undifferentiated manner. It may be associated with other congenital anomalies and may be metastatic.

CHAPTER

31

Structure and Function of the Reproductive System

OBJECTIVES

After review of this chapter, the learner will be able to:

1. Discuss the role of the hypothalamic-pituitary-ovarian axis in the regulation of reproductive structure and function.

2. Diagram normal female reproductive anatomy.

3. Describe the normal female reproductive cycle with differential hormonal levels and cellular events.

4. Diagram normal male reproductive anatomy.

5. Discuss the vascular and hormonal sequence of events required for ejaculation of motile sperm.

6. Identify the hormones necessary at puberty to promote the development of normal female breasts.

7. Describe the functions of the female breast and discuss the cyclical hormonal mediated changes in the breast tissue during the reproductive years and with pregnancy.

8. Describe the normal changes in the reproductive systems of males and females with advanced age.

LECTURE OUTLINE	INSTRUCTOR'S NOTES

Development of the Reproductive Systems
    Sexual differentiation in utero
    Puberty
The Female Reproductive System
    External genitalia
    Internal genitalia
        Vagina
        Uterus
        Fallopian tubes
        Ovaries
    Female sex hormones
        Estrogens
        Progesterone
        Androgens
    The menstrual cycle
        Phases of the menstrual cycle
        Hormonal controls
        Ovarian cycle
        Uterine phases
        Vaginal response
        Body temperature

LECTURE OUTLINE	INSTRUCTOR'S NOTES

The Male Reproductive System
    External genitalia
        Testes
        Epididymis
        Scrotum
        Penis
    Internal genitalia
    Spermatogenesis
    Male sex hormones
Structure and Function of the Breast
    The female breast
    The male breast
Aging and Reproductive Function
    Aging and the female reproductive system
    Aging and the male reproductive system

DIFFICULT CONCEPTS

Learning the Connectedness of Male and Female Reproductive Systems

When teaching male and female reproductive system anatomy and physiology, it is helpful to emphasize the homologous structures of the male and female systems. Such an approach assists students to better understand the "connectedness" of human structure and function regardless of gender.

Direct Connection Between Female Genital Ducts, Structures, and Peritoneum Lining the Pelvic Cavity

This direct connection in the female (but not in the male) is clinically important and difficult for students to appreciate. Have students complete a retrograde tracing of pathologic microorganisms through the reproductive duct systems from exterior to interior to illustrate the danger of peritonitis in the female that may result from a reproductive tract infection, such as a sexually transmitted disease.

Female Reproductive Cycles

Students often have difficulty sorting out a multiple function composite illustration, such as Figure 30-10. Encourage students to first "isolate" and then "integrate" the functions or informational items that are illustrated. You can use as an example the composite interstate highway signs that announce rest stops with different services. Availability of rest rooms, telephones, gasoline, restaurants, handicapped access, and other services is indicated by symbols. When you see such a sign, you automatically integrate the information and understand the array of services available.

Structures of the Male Genital Reproductive Ducts

Tracing sperm from point of formation in sequence through the reproductive ducts to ejaculation is as effective a learning tool as tracing blood in the cardiovascular system or air through the airways in the lungs.

CRITICAL THINKING

1. Can measuring body temperature be used as a form of birth control?

Answer: Basal body temperature undergoes biphasic changes during menstrual cycles in which ovulation occurs. During the follicular phase temperature hovers around 98° F (37° C). During the luteal phase, the average temperature increases 0.4° to 1° F (0.2–0.5° C). The increase in temperature is related to ovulation, corpus luteum formation, and increased serum progesterone levels (probably responsible for the temperature increase). Thus, an increase in basal body temperature indicates the beginning of the ovulatory phase, but not the exact time of ovulation. Measurement of body temperature is a crude form of birth control that necessitates a long period of abstinence to prevent conception.

Alterations of the Reproductive Systems Including Sexually Transmitted Diseases

OBJECTIVES

After review of this chapter, the learner will be able to:

1. Describe delayed or precocious puberty.

2. Describe the alterations in menstruation.

3. Identify the manifestations of premenstrual syndrome and at least one pathophysiologic explanation for its occurrence.

4. Discuss the various sites of infection and inflammation in the female reproductive system, including manifestations and treatments.

5. List the tumors of the female reproductive system, including treatment and prognosis of each.

6. Discuss the various sites of inflammation and infection in the male reproductive system, including manifestations and treatments.

7. Differentiate between a varicocele, hydrocele, and spermatocele.

8. Compare benign prostatic hypertrophy with prostate cancer.

9. Describe the common impairments to normal male reproductive function.

10. Differentiate between fibrocystic breast disease and breast cancer, with attention to risk factor detection, manifestations, treatment, and prognosis.

11. Identify the name, cause, and treatment for the major sexually transmitted diseases.

LECTURE OUTLINE	INSTRUCTOR'S NOTES

Alterations of Sexual Maturation
    Delayed puberty
    Precocious puberty
Disorders of the Female Reproductive System
    Hormonal and menstrual alterations
        Primary dysmenorrhea
        Primary amenorrhea
        Secondary amenorrhea
        Dysfunctional uterine bleeding
        Polycystic ovarian syndrome
        Premenstrual syndrome

Infection and inflammation
    Pelvic inflammatory disease
    Vaginitis
    Cervicitis
    Vulvitis
    Bartholinitis
Pelvic relaxation disorders
Benign growths and proliferative conditions
    Benign ovarian cysts
    Endometrial polyps
    Leiomyomas
    Adenomyosis
    Endometriosis
Cancer
    Cervical cancer
    Vaginal cancer
    Endometrial cancer
    Ovarian cancer
Sexual dysfunction
Impaired fertility
Disorders of the Male Reproductive System
    Disorders of the urethra
        Urethritis
        Urethral structures
    Disorders of the penis
        Phimosis and paraphimosis
        Peyronie disease
        Priapism
        Balanitis
        Penile cancer
    Disorders of the scrotum, testis, and epididymis
        Disorders of the scrotum
        Cryptorchidism
        Torsion of the testis
        Orchitis
        Cancer of the testis
        Impairment of sperm production and quality
        Epididymitis
    Disorders of the prostate gland
        Benign prostatic hyperplasia
        Prostatitis
        Cancer of the prostate
    Sexual dysfunction
Disorders of the Breast
    Disorders of the female breast
        Galactorrhea
        Benign breast disease (fibrocystic disease)
        Breast cancer
    Disorders of the male breast
        Gynecomastia
        Carcinoma
Sexually transmitted infections

DIFFICULT CONCEPTS

Cancer of the Reproductive Systems

The reproductive organs are common sites of cancer in both women and men. To emphasize the significance of the problem, have students construct a table starting with the highest incidence and sites of cancer, comparing women with men.

Prostatic Hypertrophy

Enlargement of the prostate from hypertrophy or carcinoma is a common cause of obstruction in urine flow. To illustrate, drill a small hole through a piece of dry sponge that is just large enough to accommodate a small diameter, soft catheter. The lumen will close quickly when the sponge is placed in water and enlarges.

Breast Cancer

Because breast cancer is the second most frequent form of cancer in women, it is important for students to understand risks for the disease. During class time have students form groups of 3 or 4 and take no more than 5 minutes to identify the risk factors for breast cancer. Tables 32-8 and 32-11 present the characteristics of benign and cancerous breast disorders. These tables are helpful in assisting students to distinguish the similarities and differences between these two classes of disorders.

CRITICAL THINKING

1. Explain why a woman who has hydrocephalus or a space-occupying lesion of the CNS may also develop primary amenorrhea.

    Answer: Hydrocephalus or space-occupying lesions of the CNS could interfere with the production or secretion of GnRH by the hypothalamus and follicle stimulating hormone (FSH) and luteinizing hormone (LH) by the pituitary gland. The ovary would not receive the necessary hormonal signals to initiate the menstrual cycle due to absent or low levels of circulating FSH and LH. Therefore, the woman would not have menses; and if this condition occurred prior to puberty, she would lack secondary sex characteristics.

2. Compare and contrast the risk factors and epidemiology of endometrial cancer and ovarian cancer.

    Answer: Women between ages 50 and 64 are at highest risk for endometrial cancer, the risk peaking at age 61. Women of Jewish ancestry have the highest incidence while women of Japanese ancestry have the lowest incidence. There may be genetic susceptibility with an autosomal dominant inheritance pattern. The risk factors associated with endometrial cancer include excessive carbohydrate and fat intake, decreased glucose tolerance, hypertension, nulliparity, early menarche, habitual abortion, hyperestrogenism, history of endometrial polyps or leiomyomas, and exposure to estrogen without progesterone.

    Ovarian cancer is the cause of 5% of all female cancer deaths. It occurs more frequently in industrialized countries and in white women. The serous tumor form of ovarian cancer occurs in women from 50 to 55 years old. The germ cell tumor form of ovarian cancer occurs in women under 30 years old. The risk factors associated with ovarian cancer include nulliparity, low parity (borne few children), smoking, asbestos and talc exposure, and estrogen replacement after menopause. The risk of ovarian cancer is slightly decreased in women who were exposed to mumps, measles, and rubella viruses before age 12 or who have significant oral contraceptive use. There appear to be no genetic susceptibility factors.

3. How would you differentiate between an enlarged testis caused by orchitis and cancer of the testis?

    Answer: Testicular enlargement occurs with both orchitis and cancer of the testes. However, in orchitis, the testis is swollen, tense, and tender, and the scrotum is red and swollen . The pain is sudden and sharp, radiating down into the involved testicle. The man with orchitis will develop a high fever, nausea, vomiting, and chills. In cancer of the testis, the enlargement may or may not be associated with dull, aching pain. Occasionally, a hydrocele may be present. If the tumor has metastasized, low back pain or cough and hemoptysis will be experienced, depending on the site of metastasis.

CHAPTER

33

Structure and Function of the Digestive System

OBJECTIVES

After review of this chapter, the learner will be able to:

1. Describe the normal structure and function of the gastrointestinal tract.

2. Identify the specific locations of absorption for the major nutrients.

3. Describe the three major reflexes of the gastrointestinal tract, including stimuli and results.

4. Describe the characteristic actions of normal intestinal flora.

5. Identify the causes of endogenous gastrointestinal infections.

6. Identify the major functions of the liver.

7. Discuss the formation and secretion of bile.

8. Discuss the exocrine functions of the pancreas, including stimuli, secretions, and outcomes.

LECTURE OUTLINE	INSTRUCTOR'S NOTES

The Gastrointestinal Tract
    Mouth and esophagus
        Salivation
        Swallowing
    The stomach
        Gastric motility
        Gastric secretion
        Phases of gastric secretion
    The small intestine
        Intestinal digestion and absorption
        Intestinal motility
    The large intestine
    Intestinal bacteria
Accessory Organs of Digestion
    The liver
        Secretion of bile
        Metabolism of bilirubin
        Vascular and hematologic functions
        Metabolism of nutrients
        Metabolic detoxification
        Storage of minerals and vitamins
    The gallbladder
    The exocrine pancreas

DIFFICULT CONCEPTS

Functional Significance of Surface Area

The plicae, villi, and microvilli are structures that increase the amount of surface area to facilitate digestion and absorption within the gastrointestinal tract. Comparing the state of Texas with the state of Colorado can help students understand the significance of structure to surface area. If the state of Colorado were pulled out flat, thus reducing the Rocky Mountains (which are like plicae and villi) to a level plane, it would be bigger than the state of Texas.

The mechanical breakdown of food also increases the surface area for exposure of food to the chemicals of digestion. For example, applesauce has a much greater surface area than a whole apple.

CRITICAL THINKING

1. Explain how the intestine moves chyme through it's length.

Answer: Neural reflexes along the length of the small intestine facilitate motility, digestion, and absorption. Motility is affected by two movements. Haustral segmentation is localized. Rhythmic contractions of circular smooth muscles divide and mix the chyme. This brings it in contact with the large absorptive surface area of the intestinal mucosa. This movement also helps propel it through the intestine. Peristalsis, the other major movement, is waves of contraction along short segments of longitudinal smooth muscle. The waves are slow enough to allow time for digestion. In the large intestine the primary movement is segmental. The movement massages the fecal mass and aids in water absorption. Propulsive movement occurs with the proximal-to-distal contraction of several haustral units. Peristaltic movements also occur and promote emptying of the colon. Reflexes also initiate propulsion in the colon.

Alterations of Digestive Function

OBJECTIVES

After review of this chapter, the learner will be able to:

1. Explain changes in structure and function that lead to diarrhea, constipation, and abdominal pain.

2. Identify the consequences of obstruction at various sites in the gastrointestinal tract.

3. Describe the causation, manifestations, treatments, outcomes, and complications of gastritis.

4. Compare the three types of peptic ulcers: duodenal, gastric, and stress ulcers.

5. Discuss the postgastrectomy syndromes as long-term complications of partial or complete gastrectomy.

6. Describe the similarities and differences between ulcerative colitis and Crohn disease.

7. Compare short-term and long-term starvation.

8. Discuss the five major complications of liver dysfunction: portal hypertension, ascites, hepatic encephalopathy, jaundice, and hepatorenal syndrome.

9. Discuss the causation, treatment options, and prognosis for alcoholic and biliary cirrhosis.

10. Discuss the similarities and differences between acute and chronic pancreatitis.

11. Discuss the risk factors, incidence, manifestations, treatment, morbidity, and mortality of the various tumors of the digestive system.

LECTURE OUTLINE	INSTRUCTOR'S NOTES

Disorders of the Gastrointestinal Tract
    Clinical manifestations of gastrointestinal
        dysfunction
        Anorexia
        Vomiting
        Constipation
        Diarrhea
        Abdominal pain
        Gastrointestinal bleeding
    Disorders of motility
        Dysphagia
        Gastroesophageal reflux
        Hiatal hernia
        Pyloric obstruction
        Intestinal obstruction
    Gastritis

LECTURE OUTLINE   **INSTRUCTOR'S NOTES**

Peptic ulcer disease
    Duodenal ulcers
    Gastric ulcers
    Stress ulcers
    Surgical treatment ulcers
    Postgastrectomy syndromes
Malabsorption syndromes
Pancreatic insufficiency
Lactase deficiency
Bile salt deficiency
Inflammatory bowel disease
    Ulcerative colitis
    Crohn disease
    Diverticular disease
Appendicitis
Vascular insufficiency
Disorders of nutrition
    Obesity
    Anorexia nervosa and bulimia
    Starvation
Disorders of the Accessory Organs of Digestion
    Clinical manifestations of liver disorders
        Portal hypertension
        Ascites
        Hepatic encephalopathy
        Jaundice
        Hepatorenal syndrome
    Disorders of the liver
        Viral hepatitis
        Fulminant hepatitis
        Cirrhosis
    Disorders of the gallbladder
        Cholelithiasis
        Cholecystitis
    Disorders of the pancreas
        Acute pancreatitis
        Chronic pancreatitis
Cancer of the Digestive System
    Cancer of the gastrointestinal tract
        Cancer of the esophagus
        Cancer of the stomach
        Cancer of the colon and rectum
    Cancer of the accessory organs of digestion
        Cancer of the liver
        Cancer of the gallbladder
        Cancer of the pancreas

DIFFICULT CONCEPTS

Motility, Secretion, and Absorption

Motility (mechanical digestion and elimination), secretion (chemical digestion), and absorption (nutrition and water and electrolyte balance) are major functions of the alimentary tract. When beginning to study the pathophysiologic consequences of disease of the alimentary system, it is helpful if students can conceptualize how structure and function are normally related. They then have a basis for understanding and predicting what alterations will occur as a result of disease, as well as accompanying clinical manifestations.

Ulcerating Lesions

Ulcerating lesions of the stomach and large intestine are significant causes of acute and chronic gastrointestinal disorders. A common feature is loss of the protective mucosal barrier along with the penetration of chemicals that cause trauma and inflammation. You can describe the loss of the protective barrier as similar to the loss of insulation in the walls of a house; the penetration of chemicals can be described as similar to the entry of cold air and the loss of warm air in the house.

CRITICAL THINKING

1. Analyze why ulcerative colitis is hypothesized to be caused by genetic and/or immune factors rather than infectious agents.

   Answer: Ulcerative colitis is an inflammatory disease. No infectious agent has been cultured or identified in anyone with ulcerative colitis. Therefore, it is increasingly unlikely that ulcerative colitis is caused by an infectious agent. The increased incidence of ulcerative colitis in identical twins and the presence of anticolon antibodies implies both genetic and immune factors. Other autoimmune diseases often occur with ulcerative colitis, such as systemic lupus erythematosus and erythema nodosum. It seems most likely that ulcerative colitis is caused by a genetic and/or immune factor.

2. Discuss the pathophysiologic relationship between cirrhosis and portal hypertension.

   Answer: Cirrhosis is an irreversible inflammatory disease of the liver which causes hepatocellular injury, diffuse fibrosis, and nodular regeneration. The progressive inflammation, fibrosis, necrosis, and scarring change the structure and function of the liver. Over time, the liver parenchyma becomes cobble-stoned or nodular. Liver functions decrease as a result of hepatocellular injury, ischemia, and necrosis. Cirrhosis may be associated with both biliary channel and venous obstruction.

   The inflammation, fibrosis, and scarring of cirrhosis creates an obstruction to the free flow of blood through the liver. Portal hypertension is the result of the obstruction causing excessively high blood pressure within the liver and portal venous system. Because blood from the gastrointestinal system and spleen must flow through the liver before returning to the heart, any obstruction in the liver creates a "back up" and increased pressure. Continued high pressure in the portal venous system causes increased use and dilation of collateral vessels (varices), splenomegaly, ascites, and hepatic encephalopathy.

Alterations of Digestive Function in Children

OBJECTIVES

After review of this chapter, the learner will be able to:

1. Describe the common congenital obstructions of the intestinal tract: cleft lip and palate, esophageal atresia, pyloric stenosis, malrotation of the intestine, meconium ileus, small bowel obstructions, congenital aganglionic megacolon, and malformations of the anus and rectum.

2. Discuss the rationale behind the infant's increased susceptibility to reflux.

3. Discuss the multiple factors implicated in failure to thrive.

4. Identify the causes and consequences of diarrhea in infants and children.

5. Define biliary atresia and discuss the damage sustained by the liver and its significance.

6. Discuss the three common metabolic disorders in children producing liver damage: galactosemia, fructosemia, and Wilson disease.

LECTURE OUTLINE	INSTRUCTOR'S NOTES

Disorders of the Gastrointestinal Tract
    Congenital impairment of motility
        Cleft lip and cleft palate
        Esophageal malformations
        Pyloric stenosis
        Malrotation
        Meconium ileus
        Meconium ileus equivalent
        Obstructions of the duodenum, jejunum, and
            ileum
        Congenital aganglionic megacolon
        Anorectal malformations
    Acquired impairment of motility
        Intussusception
        Gastroesophageal reflux
    Impairment of digestion, absorption, and nutrition
        Cystic fibrosis
        Gluten-sensitive enteropathy
        Protein energy malnutrition
        Failure to thrive
        Necrotizing enterocolitis

LECTURE OUTLINE	INSTRUCTOR'S NOTES

Diarrhea
    Acute diarrhea in children
    Chronic diarrhea in children
Disorders of the Liver
    Disorders of biliary metabolism and transport
        Physiologic jaundice of the newborn
        Biliary atresia
    Inflammatory disorders
        Hepatitis
        Cirrhosis
    Portal hypertension
        Types of portal hypertension
        Course of the disease
    Metabolic disorders

DIFFICULT CONCEPTS

Concept of Obstruction

Many disorders of the gastrointestinal and biliary tracts in children result in obstruction. One approach to assist students to understand the pathophysiology underlying clinical manifestations of obstructing lesions is to review the general consequences of obstruction in a tubular structure. Students can then generalize the process to specific structures within the gastrointestinal and biliary systems. As a demonstration, you can use a tubular balloon with a kink or twist in it to simulate an obstruction. As you continue to put air in the tube, the wall pressure increases and the lumen distends behind the obstruction. You can use your hand to grip the balloon to simulate increased peristalsis while reviewing the pathophysiology and the associated clinical manifestations.

CRITICAL THINKING

1. Both volvulus and intussusception involve structural obstructions of the ileum and/or colon. Explain the difference between these two types of obstruction. What is the result of either type of obstruction?

Answer: Volvulus is a mechanical twisting of the intestine. This twisting can be the result of malrotation. Malrotation occurs when the colon stays in the upper right quadrant. An obstructing fibrous band presses on the duodenum, allowing loops of bowel to twist on themselves. The twisting can occlude blood flow to the gut, causing ischemia and/or necrosis.

Intussusception is the telescoping or inversion of one loop of intestine into another. This usually involves the ileocecal area with invagination of the ileum into the cecum. The attaching mesentery and blood vessels are subsequently compressed between the layers of intestinal wall especially in the most folded angles. This process occurs in the direction of peristalsis, causing edema, venous stasis, and further vascular occlusion. As a result, the involved intestine becomes ischemic and/or necrotic. Untreated, intussusception is fatal.

2. Analyze why gluten-sensitive enteropathy causes steatorrhea (fatty stools) and vitamin K deficiency.

Answer: In the genetically susceptible, exposure to the protein of cereal products (gluten) causes inflammation and injury to the epithelial cells of the intestinal mucosa. This gluten-sensitive enteropathy (celiac disease or sprue) occurs primarily in the duodenum and jejunum. It is characterized by a loss of epithelial cells and microvilli greater than what the epithelium has the ability to regenerate. This leads to chronic inflammation, exudation, atrophy of villi, and decreased intestinal surface area with resulting malabsorption of nutrients. Malabsorption and exudation produce diarrhea. Steatorrhea (fatty stools) is common as a result of the malabsorption of fat in the jejunum. Vitamin K deficiency is caused by the malabsorption of fat-soluble vitamins.

CHAPTER

36

Structure and Function of the Musculoskeletal System

OBJECTIVES

After review of this chapter, the learner will be able to:

1. Identify the functions of bone.

2. Describe the formation, structure, and replacement of normal bone following a bone injury.

3. Discuss the methods by which bones are grouped and classified.

4. Discuss the methods by which joints are classified.

5. Describe the structure and function of articular cartilage.

6. Describe the structure of a motor unit.

7. Describe the cellular mechanisms of muscle contraction.

8. Discuss the factors determinant of the speed of muscle contraction.

9. Identify aging effects on the musculoskeletal system.

LECTURE OUTLINE	INSTRUCTOR'S NOTES

Structure and Function of Bones
    Elements of bone tissue
        Bone cells
        Bone matrix
        Bone minerals
    Types of bone tissue
    Characteristics of bone
    Maintenance of bone integrity
        Remodeling
        Repair
Structure and Function of Joints
    Fibrous joints
    Cartilaginous joints
    Synovial joints
        Structure of synovial joints
        Movement of synovial joints
Structure and Function of Skeletal Muscles
    Whole muscle
        Motor unit
    Components of muscle function
        Muscle contraction at the molecular level

<table>
<tr><td>

LECTURE OUTLINE

</td><td>

INSTRUCTOR'S NOTES

</td></tr>
</table>

Muscle metabolism
Muscle mechanics
Types of muscle contraction
Movement of muscle groups
Aging and the Musculoskeletal System
Aging of bones
Aging of joints
Aging of muscles

DIFFICULT CONCEPTS

Terminology of Joint Types

The multisyllabic, tongue-twisting names of some of the joint types may be made more palatable by giving the students a glossary. For example, amphi means "partial," arthro means "joint," and -osis means "condition of." Thus, amphiarthrosis means "condition of a partially movable joint."

Sliding Filaments

A set of children's toy "pick-up sticks" can be used to model the myofilaments within a myofibril. Two colors represent the two types of filament (thick and thin). Hold them arranged in an overlapping manner similar to the arrangement in a flexed, elongated sarcomere. Slide the sticks representing the thin filaments together to stimulate the shortening of a sarcomere. This demonstration usually requires practice to arrange the sticks properly.

CRITICAL THINKING

1. Discuss the process of forming new haversian systems and new trabeculae.

   Answer: Remodeling occurs in three phases and takes about four months. The goal of remodeling is to maintain the internal structure bone. Microscopic, but not gross, injury may trigger it. Cluster of bone cells, basic multicellular units, carry out remodeling. They are precursor cells of osteoclasts and osteoblasts. They are located on the free surfaces of bones and along the vascular channels, especially in marrow cavities.

   In phase I, activation, precursors in the osteoclast-forming areas of bone are triggered by a stimulus, such as a hormone, drug, vitamin, or physical stressor. In phase II, resorption, the osteoclasts form a cutting cone which gradually resorbs bone, leaving behind a resorption cavity. In longitudinal bone, the cavity follows the longitudinal axis of the haversian system; in spongy bone, it parallels the surface of the trabeculae. Phase III, formation, is the laying down of new bone, called secondary bone, by osteoblasts lining the walls of the resorption cavity. Successive layers, lamellae, in compact bone are laid down, until the resorption cavity is reduced to a narrow haversian canal around a blood vessel. In spongy bone, the same process forms new trabeculae.

Alterations of Musculoskeletal Function

OBJECTIVES

After review of this chapter, the learner will be able to:

1. Compare the types of fractures.

2. Differentiate between osteoporosis, osteomalacia, and osteomyelitis.

3. Identify the various types of musculoskeletal tumors.

4. Differentiate between inflammatory and noninflammatory joint disease and discuss a specific example of each.

5. Describe the pathophysiology of gout.

6. Identify the causes of contractures.

7. Discuss techniques to limit or decrease muscle atrophy caused by inactivity.

8. Compare disorders of the muscles produced by infection, inflammation, or metabolic abnormalities, and give a specific example of each.

9. Compare fibromyalgia and myofascial pain syndromes.

10. Describe the toxic myopathy related to alcohol abuse.

11. Describe rhabdomyosarcoma.

LECTURE OUTLINE	INSTRUCTOR'S NOTES

Musculoskeletal Injuries
    Skeletal trauma
        Fractures
        Dislocation and subluxation
    Support structures
        Sprains and strains of tendons and ligaments
        Tendinitis, epicondylitis, and bursitis
        Muscle strains
        Myoglobinuria
Disorders of Bones
    Metabolic bone diseases
        Osteoporosis
        Osteomalacia
        Paget disease
    Infectious bone disease: osteomyelitis
Disorders of the Joints
    Noninflammatory joint disease
        Types of osteoarthritis

LECTURE OUTLINE	INSTRUCTOR'S NOTES

Inflammatory joint disease
    Rheumatoid arthritis
    Ankylosing spondylitis
    Gout
Disorders of Skeletal Muscle
    Secondary muscular dysfunction
        Contractures
        Stress-induced muscle tension
        Disuse atrophy
    Fibromyalgia
    Muscle membrane abnormalities
    Myotonia
        Periodic paralysis
    Metabolic muscle diseases
        Endocrine disorders
        Diseases of energy metabolism
    Inflammatory muscle diseases: myositis
        Viral, bacterial, and parasitic myositis
        Polymyositis and dermatomyositis
    Toxic myopathies
Musculoskeletal Tumors
    Bone tumors
        Epidemiology
        Pattern of bone destruction
        Evaluation
        Types
    Muscle tumors
        Rhabdomyoma
        Rhabdomyosarcoma
        Other tumors

DIFFICULT CONCEPTS

Osteoporosis

    Clarification of bone resorption and bone formation is often necessary to understand how osteoporosis develops. Once the remodeling cycle is understood, the mechanisms causing osteoporosis become less difficult.

Rheumatoid Arthritis

    The difficulty in understanding rheumatoid arthritis is mastery of the inflammatory response. Once students are comfortable with the concepts of complement activation, immune complexes, physiologic response of the kinins and prostaglandins, and the role of neutrophils and macrophages, they can follow the pathogenesis of rheumatoid arthritis. Thus, illustrations from the normal immune and inflammation chapters can greatly facilitate their learning.

CRITICAL THINKING

1. Ms. Young has a comminuted fracture of her left tibia and fibula. Describe the stages of bone healing.

   Answer: Hematoma formation is the first stage. It is characterized by bleeding that forms a clot between the medullary canals of the bone ends and beneath the periosteum. With the necrosis of bone cells at the fracture site and the bleeding, an inflammatory reaction results. This leads to invasion of the site by inflammatory cells and osteoclasts which remove dead bone. The fracture site changes from a clot to an organized fibrin network with invasion of vascular tissue which increases blood supply to the area. Cells in the periosteum, endosteum, and bone marrow produce new bone beginning along the outer surface of the bone and moving over the fracture site. The osteoblasts synthesize a collagen matrix that becomes calcified. Remodeling occurs to remove excess callus (woven bone) and form trabeculae.

2. Ms. Shiburu has rheumatoid arthritis. What clinical signs and symptoms would be expected during her physical examination?

   Answer: Ms. Shiburu would have both systemic and local symptoms. Her systemic symptoms include fatigue, weakness, anorexia, weight loss, and generalized aching. Widespread pain, stiffness, and swelling of the joints are her primary local symptoms. Her joint involvement is symmetrical and is caused by inflammation, inflammatory exudate, and formation of new bone in the joint space. Pain is secondary to the pressure from swelling. Stiffness is caused by the synovitis. Over time, her joints will have decreased range of motion progressing to permanent joint deformity, muscle atrophy, and joint instability. She may also develop articular cartilage or subchondral bone cysts. These cysts may rupture into the joint or may develop fistula tracts to the skin surface. She may have extrasynovial rheumatoid nodules that can develop anywhere. These nodules occur most frequently in the subcutaneous skin of elbows and fingers. They may also develop in her cardiac valves, pericardium, pleura, lung parenchyma, and spleen, as well as other sites. She may also have lymphadenopathy of the nodes near her affected joints.

Alterations of Musculoskeletal Function in Children

OBJECTIVES

After review of this chapter, the learner will be able to:

1. Describe osteogenesis imperfecta.

2. Discuss the osteochondroses.

3. Describe the pathophysiology and manifestations of the muscular dystrophies.

4. Describe the most common bone tumors of childhood: osteosarcoma and Ewing sarcoma.

LECTURE OUTLINE	INSTRUCTOR'S NOTES

Congenital Defects
    Developmental dysplasia of the hip
    Deformities of the foot
Abnormal Density or Modeling of the Skeleton
    Osteogenesis imperfecta
    Scoliosis
Bone Infection: Osteomyelitis
Juvenile Rheumatic Arthritis
Avascular Diseases of the Bone: Osteochondrosis
    Legg-Calve-Perthes disease
    Osgood-Schlatter disease
Muscular Dystrophy
    Duchenne muscular dystrophy
Musculoskeletal Tumors in Children
    Bone tumors
        Osteosarcoma
        Ewing sarcoma
        Nonossifying fibroma
    Muscle tumors

DIFFICULT CONCEPTS

Classification of Muscular Dystrophies

The physiology of all types of muscular dystrophy is more or less the same. The classifications, however, are more complex because they are based on age of onset, rate of progression, distribution of muscular involvement, and inheritance patterns. Perhaps distinguishing the types of inheritance patterns gives learners the most difficulty. It is useful, therefore, to have students review normal patterns of inheritance prior to this content.

Evaluation and Treatment of Musculoskeletal Tumors in Children

Understanding the differences among plain x-ray, CT, and MRI can be facilitated by showing actual slides of each. Review of certain enzyme analyses, such as lactic dehydrogenase, and why these enzymes are elevated in children with certain musculoskeletal tumors may be necessary. Involvement by a child oncologist can help students understand how decisions are made regarding radiation, chemotherapy, immunotherapy, and surgery treatments.

CRITICAL THINKING

1. Explain the common pathophysiology of the muscular dystrophies.

   Answer: Skeletal muscle fiber degeneration is the genetic defect in all muscular dystrophies. They are familial disorders characterized by progressive, symmetric muscular weakness and atrophy of skeletal muscle groups. Each type of muscular dystrophy is distinct and probably caused by a separate defect.

   In each type there is an abnormal intracellular metabolism in the muscle fiber, resulting in a metabolic or absorption defect. Intracellularly, there are chain-forming, multiple nuclei and disruption of striation. The muscle fibers can become either hypertrophic and edematous or atrophic. As muscle fiber destruction progresses, the fibers are replaced with fat and fibrosis.

Structure, Function, and Disorders of the Integument

OBJECTIVES

After review of this chapter, the learner will be able to:

1. Describe the structure of the skin.

2. Describe the development of pressure ulcers, with attention to the risk factors for development.

3. Compare the various forms of dermatitis.

4. Compare and contrast acne vulgaris and acne rosacea.

5. Describe the skin lesions produced by the following infectious agents: Streptococcus, Staphylococcus, herpes virus, papillomavirus, tinea, and candidiasis.

6. Discuss the similarities and differences between seborrheic keratosis, keratoacanthoma, and actinic keratosis.

7. Describe the cancers of the skin, with attention to incidence, risk factors, manifestations, treatments, and prognosis.

8. Describe the depth and extent of injury for first-, second-, and third-degree burns.

9. Discuss the consequences of body fluid shifts related to burn trauma.

10. Differentiate between male and female pattern alopecia.

11. Identify the causative organisms of paronychia.

LECTURE OUTLINE	INSTRUCTOR'S NOTES

Structure and Function of the Skin
    Layers of the skin
        Dermal appendages
        Blood supply and innervation
    Clinical manifestations of skin dysfunction
        Lesions
        Pruritus
Disorders of the Skin
    Inflammatory disorders
        Allergic contact dermatitis
        Irritant contact dermatitis
        Atopic dermatitis
        Stasis dermatitis
        Seborrheic dermatitis

LECTURE OUTLINE	INSTRUCTOR'S NOTES

Papulosquamous disorders
    Psoriasis
    Pityriasis rosea
    Lichen planus
    Acne vulgaris
    Acne rosacea
    Lupus erythematosus
Vesiculobullous disorders
    Pemphigus
    Erythema multiforme
Infections
    Bacterial infections
    Viral infections
    Fungal infections
Vascular disorders
    Cutaneous vasculitis
    Urticaria
    Scleroderma
Insect bites
    Ticks
    Mosquitoes and flies
Benign tumors
    Seborrheic keratosis
    Keratoacanthoma
    Actinic keratosis
    Nevi (moles)
Cancer
    Basal cell carcinoma
    Squamous cell carcinoma
    Malignant melanoma
    Kaposi sarcoma
Thermal injury
    Burns
    Frostbite
Disorders of the Hair
    Alopecia
        Male-pattern alopecia (androcentricalopecia)
        Female-pattern alopecia
        Alopecia areata
    Hirsutism
Disorders of the Nail
    Paronychia
    Onchyomycosis

DIFFICULT CONCEPTS

Thermoregulation

A steam furnace with radiators is a good analogy for the thermoregulatory function of skin bloodflow. The furnace thermostat regulates the amount of heat from the furnace (body core) to the radiator (skin) depending on the amount of heat required to maintain normal body function.

Layers of skin from the dermis to the epidermis can be recalled more easily by using mnemonic terms. Encourage the students to make up their own as a self-study guide.

CRITICAL THINKING

1. Mr. Delgattio has psoriasis. Why would rapid epidermal proliferation cause thick, silvery, erythematous plaques?

   Answer: Psoriasis increases skin cell metabolism, causing cellular proliferation and inflammation in the epidermis and dermis. The increased metabolism raises the rate of epidermal shedding, and the new cells arrive at the surface without time for maturation and keratinization. This leads to epidermal thickening and plaque formation. The increased vascularity needed for the metabolic processes causes the erythema. The silvery color is caused by the loosely cohesive keratin.

2. Differentiate between first-, second-, and third-degree burns. Give an example of each.

   Answer: A first-degree burn is an epidermal injury in which skin functions and barrier protections are maintained. It is characterized by redness, pain, and tenderness to touch. In large first-degree burns, localized edema, chills, headache, and nausea or vomiting may occur. Blisters do not occur immediately, although they may be present after 24 hours. The skin will usually peel in 24 to 48 hours and heal within 5 days. Sunburn is an example of a first-degree burn.

   A second-degree or partial-thickness burn is an epidermal and dermal injury in which skin functions and barrier protections are absent but skin appendages are maintained. Second-degree burns can be either superficial or deep, depending on the depth of dermal injury. They both are very painful. An example of a second-degree burn is a thermal burn from a hot liquid.

   Superficial second-degree burns are characterized by the immediate development of fluid- filled blisters. The skin is red to pale ivory and moist because of the loss of the vapor barrier. The injury will heal in 21 to 28 days with the possibility of scarring, depending on genetic predisposition.

   Deep second-degree burns are characterized by either fluid-filled blisters or flat, dehydrated, tissue-papery, peeling skin. The skin is mottled with waxy white, dry areas. The injury will heal in a month or more, depending on the extent of the burn. Scarring will generally increase the longer it takes to heal and also depends on genetic predisposition.

   A third-degree or full-thickness burn is an injury that affects all layers of skin, including epidermis, dermis, and subcutaneous tissue. It may involve bone and underlying tissues. All skin appendages, skin functions, and barrier protections are lost. Blisters are rare. There is no associated pain. The skin color is cherry red, white, or black. It looks dry, thin, and papery or dry and leathery. It will heal only with skin grafting. Scarring usually occurs.

Alterations of the Integument in Children

OBJECTIVES

After review of this chapter, the learner will be able to:

1. Describe atopic and diaper dermatitis, focusing on manifestations and treatment.

2. Describe the common skin infections produced by bacteria, fungi, and viruses in children.

3. Compare the following childhood diseases: rubella, rubeola, roseola, chickenpox, shingles, and smallpox.

4. Describe how pediculosis can be spread.

5. Describe the similarities and differences between vascular skin disorders seen in children.

6. Define erythema toxicum neonatorum.

LECTURE OUTLINE	INSTRUCTOR'S NOTES

Acne Vulgaris
Dermatitis
    Atopic dermatitis
    Diaper dermatitis
Infections of the Skin
    Bacterial infections
        Impetigo contagiosum
        Staphylococcal scalded-skin syndrome
    Fungal infections
        Tinea capitis
        Tinea corporis
        Thrush
    Viral infections
        Molluscum contagiosum
        Rubella (German or 3-day measles)
        Rubeola (red measles)
        Roseola (exanthem subitum)
        Chickenpox, herpes zoster, and smallpox
Insect Bites and Parasites
    Scabies
    Pediculosis (lice)
    Fleas
    Bedbugs

LECTURE OUTLINE	INSTRUCTOR'S NOTES

Vascular Disorders
    Strawberry hemangioma
    Cavernous hemangiomas
    Salmon patches
    Port-wine stain
Other Skin Disorders
    Miliara
    Erythema toxicum neonatorum

DIFFICULT CONCEPTS

Lesion Differentiation

    One of the common difficulties in understanding skin disorders in children is comprehending the etiologies and characteristics of inflammatory lesions. A collection of slides or pictures in a 3-ring binder can be useful for learning exercises. Summaries of the lesions can be placed on the backs of the pictures or on the following slide. Guiding questions can be placed at the bottom of the picture or on the preceding slide. Students can work in small groups to work out the differentiating characteristics and related pathophysiology for each group of lesions.

CRITICAL THINKING

1. A child is diagnosed with rubella. Another child is diagnosed with rubeola. What are the differences between them?

    Answer: The child with rubella (German measles) has a viral disease that results in a red maculopapular rash on the child's face and trunk. The rash is immediately preceded by a mild fever, malaise, sore throat, and upper respiratory symptoms. Rubella's incubation period is 14 to 21 days. It resolves in 2 to 3 days without complications to the child. Infection of a pregnant woman can result in fetal congenital abnormalities.

    The child with rubeola (Measles) is also infected with a virus that results in an acute, highly contagious illness. The incubation period is 7 to 12 days. Prior to the development of a rash, the child will have a fever, cough, rhinitis, malaise, and enlarged lymph nodes. One to two days before the rash, the child will have Koplik's spots, which are pinpoint red dots with a white center in the buccal mucosa. By the third to fourth day, a purple-red (erythematous), blanching maculopapular rash will develop, which progresses to a brown, non-blanching maculopapular rash. The rash spreads from the face and upper trunk to the extremities. Measles is associated with infectious complications, including encephalitis, otitis media, and pneumonia.

TEST BANK

CHAPTER

1

Cellular Biology

Name _____

True/False

1. (T,2)   1. T   F   Prokaryotes contain no organelles and lack a distinct nucleus.

2. (F,5)   2. T   F   The function of the endoplasmic reticulum is unknown.

3. (T,4)   3. T   F   Lipids are the basic components of the plasma membrane.

4. (T,20) 4. T   F   The cell cycle can be defined as the alternation between mitosis and interphase in tissues with cellular turnover.

5. (F,24) 5. T   F   Neural tissue is the only kind of tissue that lacks cells, being composed entirely of extracellular neurons.

6. (T,2)   6. T   F   The primary functions of the cell nucleus are cell division and control of genetic information.

7. (T,5)   7. T   F   The chief function of ribosomes is to provide sites for cellular protein synthesis.

8. (T,5)   8. T   F   Lysosomes are essential for cellular digestion.

9. (T,3)   9. T   F   A primary function of the plasma membrane is to determine what a cell contains.

10. (F,6) 10. T   F   A plasma membrane is a rigid structure that does not change.

Multiple Choice

11. (c,2) 11. Which of the following best describes the cellular function of metabolic absorption?

  a. Cells can generate forces that produce motion.
  b. Cells can respond to a stimulus manifested by a wave of excitation.
  c. Cells can take in nutrients and other substances.
  d. Cells can synthesize new substances from substances they absorb.

12. (a,2) 12. Which of the following are the three components of the eukaryotic cell?

  a. cytoplasm, organelles, and plasma membrane
  b. speckles, muscle fiber, and bases
  c. neurons, acids, and synapses
  d. ribosomes, lysosomes, and chromosomes

13. (a,6)   13. The fluid mosaic model explains:

   a. how a cell membrane works.
   b. why our bodies appear to be solid.
   c. how tissue is differentiated.
   d. how sleep-wake patterns work.

14. (a,13-14) 14. Passive transport:

   a. is driven by osmosis, diffusion, or hydrostatic pressure.
   b. involves receptors that can bind with a substance being transported.
   c. is capable of transporting macromolecules.
   d. requires energy generated by the cell.
   e. none of the above.

15. (b,15)   15. In passive mediated transport:

   a. solute molecules are moved from areas of low concentration to areas of high concentra-
       tion.
   b. transport proteins move solutes through cellular membranes without expending metabolic
       energy.
   c. energy generated by the cell is always required.
   d. the process takes longer than simple diffusion.

16. (c,21)   16. Cellular reproduction is a process that:

   a. often takes months or years to complete.
   b. typically has a short interphase.
   c. results in two diploid cells called daughter cells.
   d. involves the interaction of male and female cells.

17. (e,17-18) 17. During endocytosis:

   a. a section of the plasma membrane breaks off and forms a vessicle inside the cell.
   b. transport can consist of either pinocytosis or phagocytosis.
   c. micromolecules enter the cell.
   d. lysosomal enzymes may be released.
   e. all of the above.

18. (a,18)   18. During exocytosis:

   a. macromolecules can be secreted across eukaryotic cell membranes.
   b. all substances are secreted into the cellular matrix.
   c. no repairs in the plasma membrane can take place.
   d. solute molecules flow freely into and out of the cell.
   e. all of the above.

19. (e,8)   19. Cellular receptors often bind _____ on the surface of their target cells.

   a. proteins
   b. lipids
   c. amphipathic lipids
   d. ribosomes
   e. ligands

20. (d,9)

20. Neurotransmitters are secreted during:

    a. paracrine signaling.
    b. autocrine signaling.
    c. endocrine signaling.
    d. synaptic signaling.

21. (b,12)

21. Under anaerobic conditions, the process of _____ provides energy for the cell.

    a. oxidative phosphorylation
    b. glycolysis
    c. lactolysis
    d. passive transport

22. (c,18)

22. The cellular uptake of cholesterol depends on:

    a. receptor-mediated exocytosis.
    b. antiport system.
    c. receptor-mediated endocytosis.
    d. passive transport.

23. (b,20)

23. Time during the cell cycle when DNA is synthesized is called:

    a. G_1.
    b. S.
    c. G_2.
    d. mitosis.

24. (c,20)

24. Cytokinesis is:

    a. division of nuclei.
    b. DNA replication.
    c. cytoplasmic division.
    d. nucleolus division.

25. (b,24)

25. Gating:

    a. depends on concentration of sodium ions.
    b. controls the permeability of the junctional complex.
    c. enables injured and uninjured cells to communicate.
    d. depends upon growth factors.

26. (b,4)

26. In cellular metabolism each enzyme has a high affinity for a:

    a. solute.
    b. substrate.
    c. receptor.
    d. ribosome.

27. (d,2)

27. Most of a cell's genetic information is contained in the:

    a. mitochondria.
    b. ribosome.
    c. nucleolus.
    d. nucleus.

28. (b,5)

28. The RNA-protein complex of a eukaryotic cell is the:

    a. golgi.
    b. ribosome.
    c. endoplasmic reticulum.
    d. lysosome.

29. (a,11-12)

29. The three phases of cellular catabolism are:

    a. digestion, glycolysis and oxidation, and citric acid cycle.
    b. diffusion, osmosis, and medicated transport.
    c. S phase, G phase, and M phase.
    d. metabolic absorption, respiration, and excretion.

Matching

30. (b,9)

30. ___ endocrine signaling   a. uses neurotransmitters

31. (d,9)

31. ___ paracrine signaling   b. uses hormones

32. (c,9)

32. ___ autocrine signaling   c. uses autosimulation

33. (a,9)

33. ___ synaptic signaling   d. uses local chemical mediators

Short Answer

34. List four of the seven cellular functions.

35. List the five functions of the plasma membrane.

36. How many kilocalories of chemical energy is released when 1 mole of glucose is metabolically broken down?

37. List the two functions of ATP.

38. What is the resting membrane potential in millivolts?

39. Antracellular fluid has a higher concentration of _____ ions; extracellular fluid has a

    higher concentration of _____ ions.

40. What is the difference between the absolute refractory period and the relative refractory
    period?

41. What are the two main functions of cell junctions?

42. What are the three main types of cell junctions?

43. What are the four basic tissue types?

44. What are the two types of living cells?

Short Answers

34. Movement, conductivity, metabolic absorption, secretion, excretion, respiration, reproduction (2)
35. Provides structure, provides protection, activates the cell, facilitates transport and cell-to-cell
    interaction (5)
36. 686 kcal (11)
37. 1. Stores energy
    2. Transfers energy from one molecule to another (11)
38. –270 to –85 millivolts (18)
39. Potassium; sodium (18)
40. In the absolute refractory period, the plasma membrane cannot respond to any additional stimu-
    lus. During the relative refractory period, a stronger-than-normal impulse may produce an
    action potential. (19-20)
41. 1. To hold cells together
    2. To allow small molecules to pass from cell to cell, allowing coordination of the activities
        of cells that form tissues (23)
42. 1. Desmosomes (macula adherens)
    2. Tight junctions (zonula occludens)
    3. Gap junctions (23)
43. Nerve, connective, epithelial, muscle (24)
44. Prokaryotes and eukaryotes (2)

Genes and Genetic Diseases

Name _____

True/False

1. (T,35)   1. T   F   Genes dictate the makeup of proteins.

2. (T,37)   2. T   F   The key to accurate DNA replication is complimentary base pairing.

3. (F,37)   3. T   F   RNA polymerase is the most important protein in DNA replication.

4. (F,37)   4. T   F   Silent substitutions have profound consequences on development.

5. (F,37)   5. T   F   Frameshift mutation has no impact on amino acid sequence in protein synthesis.

6. (T,39-40) 6. T   F   Missing or duplicate portions of chromosomes can be identified via karyotype.

7. (F,49)   7. T   F   If a person inherits an autosomal dominant gene for a disease, the person will definitely show the phenotype of the disease.

Multiple Choice

8. (b,36)   8. The basic components of genes are:

    a.   pentose sugar, deoxyribose, four phosphate bases.
    b.   DNA, phosphate molecule, four nitrogenous bases.
    c.   adenine, guanine, purine.
    d.   codons, oxygen, cytosine.

9. (d,37)   9. Mutation by silent substitution results in:

    a.   active disease.
    b.   silent disease.
    c.   delayed disease.
    d.   no disease.

10. (d,38)   10. The process by which RNA directs the synthesis of protein is termed:

    a.   termination sequence.
    b.   transcription.
    c.   introns.
    d.   translation.

11. (b,36)

11. The nitrogenous bases which are compoents of DNA are:

   a. amino acids.
   b. A, G, C and Ts.
   c. monosaccharides.
   d. nucleotides.

12. (c,36)

12. The genetic code is:

   a. organism specific.
   b. unknown.
   c. universal.
   d. evolving.

13. (c,39)

13. An ordered photographic display of a set of chromosomes from a single cell is a:

   a. metaphase spread.
   b. autosomal spread.
   c. karyotype.
   d. anaphase spread.

14. (b,41)

14. An error in which homologous chromosomes fail to separate during meiosis is termed:

   a. aneuploidy.
   b. nondisjunction.
   c. polyploidy.
   d. anaplasia.

15. (d,40)

15. Many spontaneous abortions occur because of:

   a. chromosome aberrations.
   b. tetraploidy.
   c. triploidy.
   d. all of the above.

16. (b,41)

16. _____ is a condition in which only an extra portion of a chromosome is present in each cell.

   a. Fragmented trisomy
   b. Partial trisomy
   c. Translocated trisomy
   d. Down syndrome

17. (a,40)

17. _____ cells do not contain a multiple of 23 chromosomes.

   a. Aneuploid
   b. Mutant
   c. Diploid
   d. Polyploid

18. (d,40)

18. A cell containing a multiple of the normal number of chromosomes is a/an _____ cell.

   a. aneuploid
   b. mosaic
   c. trisomy
   d. euploid

19. (b,40)

19. Nearly all triploid fetuses are:

    a.   geniuses.
    b.   aborted or stillborn.
    c.   mentally retarded.
    d.   short and obese.

20. (b,41)

20. If a person is a chromosomal mosaic, the person may:

    a.   be a carrier of the genetic disease.
    b.   have a mild form of the genetic disease.
    c.   have two genetic diseases.
    d.   be sterile as a result of the genetic disease.

21. (c,42)

21. The most common cause of Down syndrome is:

    a.   paternal nondisjunction.
    b.   maternal translocations.
    c.   maternal nondisjunction.
    d.   paternal translocations.

22. (c,44)

22. Jane Brown, age 13, has a karyotype that reveals an absent homologous X chromosome with only a single X chromosome present. Her condition is called:

    a.   Down syndrome.
    b.   Criduchat syndrome.
    c.   Turner syndrome.
    d.   Edward syndrome.

23. (d,45)

23. Based on Jane Brown's condition, which of the following would you expect to see clinically?

    a.   possibly some impairment of mathematical reasoning ability
    b.   sterility
    c.   widely spaced nipples
    d.   all of the above

24. (b,44)

24. An XXY person has the genetic disorder called:

    a.   Turner syndrome.
    b.   Klinefelter syndrome.
    c.   Down syndrome.
    d.   none of the above.

25. (a,45)

25. Characteristic signs of Klinefelter syndrome include:

    a.   high-pitched voice.
    b.   female genitalia.
    c.   dense body hair.
    d.   absent breast development.

26. (b,46)

26. The second most commonly recognized genetic cause of mental retardation is:

    a.   Down syndrome.
    b.   fragile X syndrome.
    c.   Klinefelter syndrome.
    d.   Turner syndrome.

27. (b,51)

27. People who have neurofibromatosis will show varying degrees of the disease; this is because of the genetic principle of:

    a.   penetrance.
    b.   expressivity.
    c.   dominance.
    d.   recessiveness.

28. (d,52)

28. Cystic fibrosis is caused by an _____ gene.

    a.   X-linked dominant
    b.   X-linked recessive
    c.   autosomal dominant
    d.   autosomal recessive

29. (c,53)

29. A genetically normal male is always _____ for genes on the X chromosome.

    a.   homozygous
    b.   heterozygous
    c.   hemizygous

30. (b,55)

30. Which of the following disorders has a sex-linked mode of inheritance?

    a.   cat-cry syndrome
    b.   (DMD) Duchenne muscular dystrophy
    c.   cystic fibrosis
    d.   Down syndrome

31. (c,52)

31. If a boy inherits a disease that is autosomal recessive, he inherited it from his:

    a.   father.
    b.   mother.
    c.   father and mother.

32. (a,53)

32. _____ are affected most often by X-linked recessive genes.

    a.   Males
    b.   Females
    c.   Neither males nor females

33. (b,54)

33. If a boy inherits Duchenne muscular dystrophy, he inherited it from his:

    a.   father.
    b.   mother.
    c.   mother and father.

34. (d,54)

34. Joey, age 9, is admitted to the pediatric ward with Duchenne muscular dystrophy. He inherited this condition through a:

    a.   sex-linked dominant trait.
    b.   sex-influenced trait.
    c.   sex-limited trait.
    d.   sex-linked recessive trait.

35. If Jane Brown's problem is multifactorial or polygenic, which of the following must occur before the disease is expressed?

    a.   somatic cell hybridization
    b.   threshold liability
    c.   empiric risks
    d.   in situ hybridization

Matching

36. Rh disease

    a. chromosome pair 1

37. Familial colon cancer

    b. chromosome pair 21

38. Down syndrome

    c. chromosome pair XY

39. Cystic fibrosis

    d. chromosome pair 7

40. Hemophilia

    e. chromosome pair 2

Short Answer

41. What are neucleotides composed of?

42. List three mutations and describe them.

43. RNA mediates what two basic processes in protein formation in cytoplasm?

44. What are claustogens?

45. Name and describe Mendel's two basic laws of inheritance.

Short Answers

41. 1 Deoxyribase molecule, one phosphate group, one base (36)
42. 1. Silent substitution—no change in the amino acids
    2. Base pair substitution—one base pair replaced by another
    3. Framework mutation—the insertion or deletion of one or more base pairs of the DNA molecule
    4. Spontaneous mutations—those occurring in the absence of exposure to a mutagen (37)
43. Transcription and translation (37)
44. They are harmful agents, such as ionizing radiation, viral infections, and chemicals, that contribute to chromosomal breakage increases. (45)
45. 1. Principle of segregation—homologous genes separate from another during reproduction, and each reproductive cell carries only one homologous gene.
    2. Principle of independent assortment—the heredity transmission of one gene does not affect the transmission of another. (48)

Altered Cellular and Tissue Biology

Name _____

True/False

1. (F,66)

1. T   F   All cells are capable of hyperplasia.

2. (F,66)

2. T   F   Dysplasia is a common type of normal cellular adaptation.

3. (T,66)

3. T   F   Hypertrophy and hyperplasia often occur together.

4. (F,65)

4. T   F   Atrophy most often occurs in hepatocytes, spleen cells, and the lens of the eye.

5. (T,66)

5. T   F   A biopsy of epithelial cells in Mr. Simon's airway (bronchial) reveals that the normal columnar ciliated cells have been replaced by stratified squamous epithelial cells. Mr. Simon is correctly told that this process could be reversed if he quits smoking.

6. (F,66)

6. T   F   The type of cellular adaptation occurring in Mr. Simon's airway is called atrophy.

7. (T,67)

7. T   F   Physical and mechanical factors can cause cellular injury.

8. (T,65)

8. T   F   Hypertrophy of the remaining kidney is a normal cellular adaptation following removal of one kidney.

9. (T,68)

9. T   F   The most common cause of hypoxia is ischemia.

Multiple Choice

10. (d,69)

10. Free radicals cause cellular injury by:

   a.   stopping protein synthesis.
   b.   disrupting lysosomal membranes.
   c.   transforming cells into cancerous cells.
   d.   forming injurious chemical bonds.

11. (c,90)

11. Liquefactive necrosis occurs in the brain because:

   a.   debris is not digested by hydrolases.
   b.   of protein denaturation (gelatinous to opaque state).
   c.   it is rich in hydrolytic enzymes and lipids.
   d.   ischemia results in chemical injury.

12. (c,98)

12. Postmortem reduction of body temperature is called:

    a. rigor mortis.
    b. livor mortis.
    c. algor mortis.
    d. mortor mortis.

13. (e,69)

13. Consequences of ischemia include:

    a. decreased production of ATP.
    b. increased intracellular lactate.
    c. decreased protein synthesis.
    d. a and c.
    e. a, b, and c.

14. (e,72)

14. Biologically relevant free radicals include:

    a. reactive oxygen species.
    b. nitric oxide.
    c. hydrogen peroxide.
    d. a and b.
    e. a, b, and c.

15. (d,72-73)

15. In chemical injury, damage by free radicals occurs via:

    a. lipid peroxidation.
    b. direct toxicity.
    c. phagocytosis.
    d. a and b.
    e. a, b, and c.

16. (a,92)

16. In distinguishing aging from diseases:

    a. it is difficult to tell the difference because both processes are believed to result from cell injury.
    b. it is easy to tell normal processes from abnormal processes.
    c. disease, unlike aging, has a genetic component.
    d. aging is defined as exceeding life expectancy but not maximal life span.

17. (b,66)

17. The mammary glands enlarge during pregnancy primarily as a consequence of:

    a. compensatory hyperplasia.
    b. hormonal hyperplasia.
    c. hormonal anaplasia.
    d. hormonal dysplasia.

18. (d,67)

18. The extent of injury a cell may incur from a given insult is profoundly influenced by the cell's:

    a. type.
    b. adaptive processes.
    c. metabolic state.
    d. all of the above.

19. (a,67-73)

19. Cellular injury can be caused by:

   a. ischemia, lead, and bacteria.
   b. atrophy, water, and glycogen.
   c. melanin, hyperplasia, and proteins.
   d. pigments, calcium, and lipids.

20. (e,87)

20. Hemosiderosis may be an indication of:

   a. excessive dietary iron.
   b. excessive alcohol intake.
   c. a genetic disorder of iron metabolism.
   d. a genetic disorder of erythrocyte production.
   e. possibly any of these.

21. (e,88)

21. Metastatic calcification may be caused by:

   a. kidney disease.
   b. excessive vitamin D.
   c. bone disease.
   d. hormonal disease.
   e. any of the above.

22. (b, 91)

22. A type of necrosis often associated with pulmonary tuberculosis is:

   a. fat.
   b. caseous.
   c. liquefactive.
   d. gangrenous.
   e. all of the above.

23. (a,65)

23. Muscular hypertrophy may involve an increase in muscle cell:

   a. number.
   b. size.
   c. vacuoles.
   d. lipofuscin.

24. (b,65)

24. When the heart's workload increases, myocardial cells:

   a. divide.
   b. enlarge.
   c. increase in number.
   d. undergo metaplasia.

25. (d,70)

25. After the removal of one kidney, the remaining kidney adapts by:

   a. hypertrophy.
   b. hyperplasia.
   c. dysplasia.
   d. a and b.
   e. a, b, and c.

26. (a,66)

26. After ovulation, the uterine endometrial cells divide under the influence of estrogen. This is an example of:

    a.   hormonal hyperplasia.
    b.   hormonal dysplasia.
    c.   hormonal hypertrophy.
    d.   none of the above.

27. (b,66)

27. Atypical hyperplasia is also known as:

    a.   metaplasia.
    b.   dysplasia.
    c.   hypertrophy.
    d.   none of the above.

28. (b,66)

28. The replacement of columnar epithelial cells in the bronchi with squamous epithelial cells is an example of:

    a.   dysplasia.
    b.   metaplasia.
    c.   hypertrophy.
    d.   atrophy.
    e.   none of the above.

29. (d,66)

29. _____ is the abnormal proliferation of cells, in response to excessive hormonal stimulation.

    a.   Dysplasia
    b.   Pathologic dysplasia
    c.   Hyperplasia
    d.   Pathologic hyperplasia

30. (c,66)

30. Removal of part of the liver leads to _____ of the remaining liver cells.

    a.   dysplasia
    b.   metaplasia
    c.   compensatory hyperplasia
    d.   compensatory dysplasia

31. (d,88)

31. An important common pathway in many causes of cell death involves:

    a.   sodium
    b.   potassium
    c.   magnesium
    d.   calcium

32. (a,83)

32. Intracellular deposits of water, lipids, proteins, and pigments are all examples of:

    a.   accumulations.
    b.   aging changes.
    c.   chemical injury.
    d.   exogenous agents.

33. (c,66)	33. Cellular _____ is strongly associated with cancer.

    a.   metaplasia
    b.   atrophy
    c.   dysplasia
    d.   hypertrophy

34. (d,87)   34. _____ is a pigment that causes jaundice when high levels of it are present.

    a.   Hemosiderin
    b.   Melanin
    c.   Lipofuscin
    d.   Bilirubin

Matching: *Gunshot wounds*

35. (b,80)	35. ____ stripping	a. contact range entrance wounds
36. (a,80)	36. ____ muzzle imprint	b. intermediate range entrance wounds
37. (c,81)	37. ____ varying hole sizes	c. distant range entrance wound
38. (c,81)	38. ____ rim of abrasion	
39. (a,80)	39. ____ blow back	
40. (b,80)	40. ____ tattooing	

Matching: *Theories of aging*

41. (e,96)	41. ____ somatic mutation hypothesis	a. errors in transcription and translation eventually lead to cell death
42. (a,96)	42. ____ catastrophic theory	
43. (d,96)	43. ____ neuroendocrine theory	b. aging results from decreased ability to fight disease
44. (f,97)	44. ____ wear and tear theory	c. each cell has a finite life span
45. (c,96)	45. ____ programmed aging theory	d. genetic program for aging is encoded in the brain
46. (b,96)	46. ____ immune theory	e. aging is a result of DNA damage
		f. damages accumulate with time

Short Answer

47. What are the three common forms of cell injury?

48. List the three ways free radicals may be initiated within cells.

49. Why do most lead poisonings occur in children?

50. List three blunt force injuries.

Short Answers

47. 1. Hypoxic injury
    2. Free radicals and reactive oxygen species injury
    3. Chemical injury (67)
48. 1. The absorption of extreme energy sources
    2. Endogenous reactions when oxygen is reduced to water created by systems involved in electron and oxygen transport
    3. Enzymatic metabolism of exogenous chemicals or drugs (69-70)
49. 1. Lead-based paint has a sweet taste.
    2. Children absorb lead more readily from their intestinal tract. (73)
50. 1. Contusion
    2. Hematoma
    3. Closed fracture (78-79)

Fluids and Electrolytes, Acids and Bases

Name _____

True/False

1. (T,114)

1. T F   Both hypokalemia and hyperkalemia can cause muscle weakness.

2. (T,114)

2. T F   Nasogastric suctioning can cause hypokalemia.

3. (T,116)

3. T F   Insulin can be given to correct for hyperkalemia.

4. (T,120)

4. T F   Diarrhea can result in metabolic acidosis.

5. (T,118)

5. T F   Proteins are an important intracellular buffer.

6. (T,120)

6. T F   Renal failure may result in metabolic acidosis.

Multiple Choice

7. (b,118-119)

7. Which of the following buffer pairs is considered the major plasma buffering system?

    a. $NaCl/KPO_4$
    b. HCO_3/H_2CO_3
    c. HPO_4/H_2PO_4
    d. NH_3/NH_4

8. (a,118)

8. Physiologic pH is maintained around 7.4 because carbonic acid and bicarbonate exist in a ratio of:

    a.   20/1.
    b.   1/20.
    c.   10/2.
    d.   10/5.

9. (d,120)

9. Causes of metabolic alkalosis include:

    a.   an increase in noncarbonic acids.
    b.   hyperaldosteronism.
    c.   an excess loss of Cl.
    d.   b and c.
    e.   a, b, and c.

10. (c,121)

10. Causes of respiratory acidosis include:

   a. vomiting.
   b. kyphoscoliosis.
   c. pneumonia.
   d. b and c.
   e. a, b, and c.

11. (b,116)

11. Metabolic acidosis is often accompanied by:

   a. hypokalemia.
   b. hyperkalemia.
   c. hypernatremia.
   d. hyponatremia.

12. (b,104)

12. The normal male has a daily water intake and output of about:

   a. 1 liter.
   b. 3 liters.
   c. 5 liters.
   d. 0.5 liter.

13. (a,105)

13. Water movement between the intracellular fluid compartment and the extracellular compartment is according to:

   a. osmotic forces.
   b. plasma oncotic pressure.
   c. antidiuretic hormone.
   d. buffer systems.

14. (b,107-108)

14. Secretion of ADH is stimulated by:

   a. a decrease in serum sodium and serum potassium.
   b. nerve endings sensitive to changes in volume and pressure.
   c. an increase in glomerular filtration rate.
   d. generalized edema.

15. (c,121)

15. Tony Buffer, age 54, has a long history of smoking. He decides to have lung and blood studies done because he's very tired, short of breath, and just doesn't feel good. His blood gases reveal the following findings: decreased pH, increased CO_2, and normal HCO_3. Tony's condition may be:

   a. respiratory alkalosis.
   b. metabolic acidosis.
   c. respiratory acidosis.
   d. metabolic alkalosis.

16. (e,105-106)

16. Edema may be caused by:

   a. increasing capillary permeability.
   b. removing lymphatic tissue.
   c. reducing plasma proteins.
   d. increasing interstitial proteins.
   e. any of the above.

17. (a,107)

17. Edema due to third spacing may result in:
    a. dehydration.
    b. lymphedema.
    c. increased urine output.
    d. decreased pulse rate.

18. (d,107)

18. Water balance is closely related to _____ balance.

    a. potassium
    b. chloride
    c. bicarbonate
    d. sodium

19. (c,107)

19. In addition to thirst, osmoreceptors may be stimulated when:

    a. ADH decreases.
    b. blood volume increases.
    c. serum osmolality increases.
    d. serum sodium decreases.

20. (d,108)

20. The secretion of aldosterone is influenced by:

    a. serum sodium levels.
    b. serum potassium levels.
    c. blood volume.
    d. all of the above.

21. (b,111)

21. Hypernatremia is usually caused by

    a. hepatitis.
    b. Cushing syndrome.
    c. trauma to the hypothalamus.
    d. pancreatitis.

22. (a,116)

22. The electrocardiogram shows tall T waves in:

    a. hyperkalemia.
    b. hypokalemia.
    c. hypernatremia.
    d. hyponatremia.

23. (b,114)

23. Treatment of pernicious anemia with vitamin B or folate may precipitate:

    a. hyperkalemia.
    b. hypokalemia.
    c. hypernatremia.
    d. hyponatremia.

24. (b,104)

24. From birth to adulthood, the percentage of total body water:

    a. increases.
    b. decreases.
    c. is unchanged.
    d. fluctuates widely.

25. (a,109)   25. _____ alterations occur when changes in TBW are accompanied by proportional changes in electrolytes.

a. Isotonic
b. Hypertonic
c. Hypotonic
d. None of the above

Matching

26. (a,108)   26. ___   90% of ECF cations   a. sodium

27. (a,108)   27. ___   natriurectic hormone promotes excretion   b. chloride

28. (b,108)   28. ___   inversely related to HCO$_3$ concentration   c. potassium

29. (c,113)   29. ___   major cation in intracellular spaces   d. magnesium

30. (b,108)   30. ___   major anion in extracellular spaces   e. calcium

31. (c,113)   31. ___   major determinant of resting membrane potential

32. (e,117)   32. ___   major cation for structure of bones and teeth

33. (d,117)   33. ___   60% stored in muscle and bone

34. (e,117)   34. ___   vitamin D facilitates absorption

35. (d,117)   35. ___   important for smooth muscle contraction and relaxation

Short Answer

36. What causes the decrease in total body water in the elderly?

37. Net filtration = _____ – _____.

38. Give an example of localized and of generalized edema.

39. What is the difference between dehydration and pure water deficit?

40. Body acids exist in what two forms? Describe them.

Short Answers

36. 1.   Increased body fat
    2.   Decreased muscle mass
    3.   Reduced ability to regulate sodium and water balance (104)
37. Force favoring filtration – forces opposing filtration (105)
38. Localized: Swelling at a trauma site, cerebral edema, pulmonary edema, pleural effusion, pericardial effusion, ascites
    Generalized: Dependant edema, third spacing in severe burns, allergic reaction (106-107)
39. Dehydration describes water and sodium loss. In pure water deficit, only water is lost. (111)
40. Volatile—can be eliminated through the lungs as CO_2 gas.
    Novolatile—cannot be excreted as CO_2; must be eliminated through the kidneys. (116)

CHAPTER

5

Immunity

Name _____

True/False

1. (F,128)

1. T   F   If a person is given an injection to provide passive acquired immunity, the person will have lifelong immunity.

2. (F,128)

2. T   F   Active acquired immunity does not involve the host's immune response.

3. (T,140)

3. T   F   Opsonization is a process which renders bacteria more susceptible to phagocytosis.

4. (F,125)

4. T   F   Most bacteria cannot live on the skin surface because of its alkalitic nature.

Multiple Choice

5. (b,128)

5. Acquired immunity is gained:

    a.   in utero.
    b.   after birth.
    c.   via injection of specific antibodies.
    d.   in adulthood.

6. (a,128)

6. If a person has innate resistance to a disease, the person has _____ immunity.

    a.   natural
    b.   native
    c.   active acquired
    d.   passive
    e.   cell-mediated

7. (b,128)

7. The immunoglobin that crosses the placenta confers _____ immunity to the fetus.

    a.   active acquired
    b.   passive acquired
    c.   inate
    d.   cell-mediated

8. (b,129)

8. The predominant antibody of a typical primary immune response is:

    a. IgG.
    b. IgM.
    c. IgA.
    d. IgD.
    e. IgE.

9. (c,129)

9. If a person is given antigen X and is later given antigen Y, a _____ response to antigen Y will result.

    a. secondary
    b. anamnestic
    c. primary
    d. none of the above

10. (a,129)

10. The _____ response protects against recurrent varicella infections.

    a. secondary
    b. primary
    c. neither provides protection

11. (a,129)

11. When a person is given an attenuated antigen, the antigen is:

    a. alive, but less infectious.
    b. mutated, but highly infectious.
    c. normal, but not infectious.
    d. inactive, but infectious.

12. (a,132)

12. A molecule that can induce the formation of antibodies is:

    a. antigen.
    b. hapten.
    c. immunogen.
    d. none of the above.

13. (e,135)

13. Both B and T cells are originially derived from cells of the:

    a. pancreas.
    b. gut associated lymphoid tissue.
    c. lymph nodes.
    d. thymus.
    e. bone marrow.

14. (c,129)

14. The immune response can be subdivided into two responses, humoral and cell-mediated. These two mechanisms include all of the following *except*:

    a. B cells.
    b. T cells.
    c. bradykinin.
    d. antibodies.

15. (d,128)

15. In what situation would the normal immune response be harmful?

   a. following organ transplant
   b. in an allergic reaction
   c. during infections
   d. a and b
   e. a, b, and c

16. (a,127)

16. Myeloid lineage does not produce:

   a. T-cells.
   b. mast cells.
   c. platelets.
   d. macrophages.

17. (c,129)

17. Which of the following is responsible for cell-mediated imunity?

   a. IgM
   b. IgG
   c. T cells
   d. B cells

18. (b,132)

18. The most important determinant of immune system activation is:

   a. size.
   b. foreignness.
   c. complexity.
   d. quantity.

19. (c,133)

19. If a person has type O blood, she is likely to have high titers (levels) of anti _____ antibodies.

   a. A only
   b. B only
   c. A and B
   d. O

20. (d,133)

20. Because of a severe blood loss, Marc is in need of a transfusion. His blood type is determined to be type AB. What blood type could Marc receive?

   a. type O
   b. type A
   c. type B
   d. all of the above

21. (d,134)

21. When a mature B-cell receptor binds to an antigen, the following occurs:

   a. production of mature immunoglobulin-secreting plasma cells
   b. development of antigenic receptors
   c. production of long-lived memory cells
   d. a and c
   e. a, b, and c

22. (a,137)

22. The most abundant class of antibody in the serum is:

   a. IgG.
   b. IgM.
   c. IgA.
   d. IgD.
   e. IgE .

23. (d,137-139)

23. When an antibody binds to its appropriate antigen:

   a. agglutination may occur.
   b. neutralization may occur.
   c. precipitation may occur.
   d. all of the above.
   e. none of the above.

24. (a,134)

24. The five classes of immunoglobulins are classified by all of the following *except*:

   a. hormonal differences.
   b. antigenic differences.
   c. structural differences.
   d. functional differences.

25. (a,140)

25. Maternal Ig _____ is the major antibody found in fetal blood.

   a. G
   b. M
   c. A
   d. D
   e. E

26. (b,141)

26. Which of the following characteristics is shared by both the secretory and systemic immune systems?

   a. lymphocytic paths of migration
   b. neutralization following antigen-antibody binding
   c. timing of response
   d. location of response

27. (c,142)

27. The cell-mediated immune response is characterized by (choose the most complete answer):

   a. cytotoxicity and memory only.
   b. cytotoxicity, memory, and delayed hypersensitivity only.
   c. memory, cytotoxicity, control, and delayed hypersensitivity.
   d. the secondary immune response only.

28. (a,140)

28. Monoclonal antibodies are better than conventional antisera because:

   a. a single antibody is generated rather than a mixture of antibodies.
   b. they have multiple binding affinities.
   c. they are polyclonal.
   d. they are less expensive.

29. (d,141)

29. The primary role of secretory IgA is to prevent infections in:

a. blood vessels.
b. kidneys.
c. lungs.
d. mucous membranes.

30. (c,140)

30. Pure monoclonal antibodies are produced:

a. by T lymphocytes.
b. by bone marrow.
c. by laboratories.
d. by fetuses.

31. (c,148)

31. A 5-month-old child is admitted to the hospital with recurring respiratory infections. A possible cause of this condition is:

a. hypergammaglobulinemia.
b. increased maternal IgG.
c. immune insufficiency.
d. decreased maternal antibody breakdown, resulting in hyposensitivity.

32. (a,143)

32. Increased age may cause which of the following?

a. decreased T-cell function
b. decreased production of antibodies against self-antigens
c. decreased production of autoantibodies
d. decreased numbers of circulating immune complexes

Matching

33. (b,144)

33. ____ lymphokine that defends against tumor cell growth and viruses

a. interleukins

b. interferon

34. (e,144)

34. ____ produced in response to inflammation, tumor growth, and cellular differentiation

c. tumor necrosis factor

35. (c,144)

35. ____ produced by macrophages, T-cells, and NK cells in response to inflammation, tumor

d. colony stimulating factors

36. (d,144)

36. ____ causes differentiation in blood cells

e. transforming growth factors

37. (a,144)

37. ____ biochemical messengers sent from one leukocyte to another

Short Answer

38. Describe the clonal selection theory.

39. List the four functions of antibiotics.

40. Why are monoclonal antibodies better than conventional antisera?

Short Answers

38. It postulates that a large number of B cells with plasma membrane receptors for all potential antigenic determinants are spontaneously generated during fetal life, independant of the presence of an antigen. Each B cell responds to only one specific antigen. When the immunocompetent B cells encounter an antigen for the first time, those with specific membrane antibody receptors complimentary to that antigen's determinant sites are stimulated to proliferate. (134)

39. 1. Neutralize bacterial toxins
    2. Neutralize viruses
    3. Opsonize bacteria
    4. Activate components of the inflammatory response (137)

40. 1. A single antibody of known antigenic specificity is generated rather than a mixture of different antibodies.
    2. Monoclonal antibodies have a single, constant binding affinity.
    3. Monoclonal antibodies can be diluted to a constant titer because the actual antibody concentration is known.
    4. The antibody can be easily purified to homogeneity. (140)

Inflammation

Name _____

True/False

1. (T,164)

2. (F,166)

3. (T,151)

4. (T,171)

5. (F,154)

1. T F Several types of bacteria can thrive inside macrophages.

2. T F Eosinophils phagocytose parasites.

3. T F Inflammation is a biochemical and cellular process that occurs in vascularized tissue.

4. T F Resolution is best defined as the restoration of original structure and physiologic function.

5. T F Chemotactic factors are released during chronic inflammation.

Multiple Choice

6. (c,152)

6. Which of the following shows a correct sequence in the inflammatory process?

   a. granuloma formation, acute inflammation, chronic inflammation
   b. chronic inflammation, granuloma formation, healing
   c. acute inflammation, chronic inflammation, granuloma formation
   d. chronic inflammation, acute inflammation, granuloma formation

7. (d,151)

7. Characteristics of inflammation include all of the following *except*:

   a. pain.
   b. localized loss of function.
   c. swelling.
   d. pallor.

8. (d,152)

8. An acute inflammatory response is triggered by:

   a. cellular injury.
   b. microorganisms.
   c. cells from dead parasites.
   d. all of the above.

9. (d,152)

9. Which of the following is *not* part of the acute inflammatory response?

   a. neutrophils
   b. mast cells
   c. monocytes
   d. granulomas

10. (d,152)

10. Cells in the blood that probably function in the same way as tissue mast cells are:

    a. neutrophils.
    b. eosinophils.
    c. macrophages.
    d. basophils.

11. (a,154)

11. _____ is directional movement of cells along a chemical gradient formed by a chemotactic factor.

    a. Chemotaxis
    b. Immigration
    c. Extravasion
    d. Degranulation

12. (d,166)

12. Eosinophils function in all of the following ways *except*:

    a. dissolving surface membranes of parasites.
    b. acting as biochemical mediators.
    c. controlling the effects of serotonin and histamine.
    d. being the first phagocyte cells to arrive at site of inflammation.

13. (a,152)

13. The mast cell, a major activator of inflammation, initiates the inflammatory response by:

    a. degranulation and mediator synthesis.
    b. degranulation and endocytosis.
    c. degranulation and cytokinesis.
    d. degranulation and hemolysis.

14. (a,151)

14. The early facilitators of inflammation are collectively known as:

    a. exudate.
    b. platelets.
    c. kinins.
    d. complement.

15. (a,156)

15. The complement system, clotting system, and kinin system share which of the following characteristics?

    a. proenzyme activation
    b. phagocytosis initiation
    c. granulocyte production
    d. interferon inhibition

16. (a,155)

16. _____ block(s) the synthesis of prostaglandins, thereby inhibiting some aspects of the acute inflammatory response.

    a. Aspirin
    b. Morphine
    c. Vitamin K
    d. Penicillin

17. (b,157)

17. _____ activates the classic pathway of the complement system.

   a. Histamine
   b. Antigen-antibody complex
   c. Leukotriene
   d. Prostaglandins

18. (d,157)

18. Activation of the complement system produces compounds which:

   a. opsonize bacteria.
   b. decrease chemotaxis of leukocytes.
   c. induce mast cell degranulation.
   d. a and c.
   e. a, b, and c.

19. (b,158)

19. The _____ system is a plasma protein system that forms a fibrinous exudate at an inflamed site to trap exudates, microbes, and foreign bodies.

   a. complement
   b. coagulation
   c. kinin
   d. none of the above

20. (d,159)

20. Bradykinin is involved in all of the following *except*:

   a. inducing pain.
   b. inducing smooth muscle contraction.
   c. increasing vascular permeability.
   d. increasing degradation of prostaglandins.

21. (c,158)

21. In the clotting cascade, the intrinsic and the extrinsic pathways converge at:

   a. C5.
   b. Hageman factor.
   c. factor X.
   d. collagen.

22. (b,159)

22. Which of the following is a correct sequence in the clotting cascade?

   a. fibrin, thrombin, fibrinogen
   b. xa, thrombin, fibrin
   c. thrombin, xa, fibrin
   d. fibrinogen, xa, fibrin

23. (d,154)

23. When histamine and seratonin are released:

   a. capillaries constrict.
   b. vascular permeability decreases.
   c. large vessel musculature dilates.
   d. microcirculation improves.

24. (c,160)

24. Frequently H_1 and H_2 receptors are located on the same cells and act in a/an _____ fashion.

   a. synergistic
   b. additive
   c. antagonistic
   d. agonistic

25. (a,161)   25. Before becoming activated, plasmin exist as:

a. plasminogen.
b. bradykinin.
c. leukotriene.
d. prothrombin.
e. Hageman factor.

26. (b,162)   26. _____ are cytoplasmic fragments that function to stop bleeding.

a. Complements
b. Platelets
c. Neutrophils
d. Eosinophils
e. PAFs

27. (e,163)   27. Neutrophils and macrophages differ in:

a. the length of time they remain active.
b. lysosomal contents.
c. arrival time at the site of inflammation.
d. factors that attract them.
e. all of the above.

28. (a,163)   28. The phagocyte's role begins when the inflammatory response causes it to stick avidly to capillary walls in a process called:

a. pavementing.
b. extravation.
c. diapedesis.
d. emigration.

29. (c,163)   29. Which of the following indicates a correct sequence in phagocytosis?

a. recognition, fusion, engulfment, destruction
b. engulfment, recognition, fusion, destruction
c. recognition, engulfment, fusion, destruction
d. engulfment, fusion, recognition, destruction

30. (b,164)   30. _____ are the largest normal blood cells.

a. Neutrophils
b. Monocytes
c. Basophils
d. Platelets

31. (a,164)   31. _____ are the predominant phagocytic cell early in the inflammatory response.

a. Neutrophils
b. Monocytes
c. Macrophages
d. Eosinophils

32. (b,164)

32. Which of the following is a true statement?

    a. Eosinophils are first to arrive at the inflammatory site.
    b. Neutrophils are incapable of cell division.
    c. Macrophages provide a short-term defense against infectious agents.
    d. all of the above

33. (d,154)

33. Mast cell degranulation is *not* stimulated by:

    a. ultraviolet light.
    b. snake venom.
    c. mechanical trauma.
    d. high altitudes.

34. (a,169)

34. One systemic manifestation of the acute inflammatory response is fever, which is produced by:

    a. IL-1 acting directly on the hypothalamus.
    b. bacterial edotorin acting on the thalamus.
    c. antigen-antibody complexes acting directly at the cerebellum.
    d. the combination of bacterial endotoxins and antigen-antibody complexes acting directly on the hypothalamus.

35. (a,169)

35. The main difference between acute and chronic inflammation is:

    a. duration.
    b. chemotaxic involvement.
    c. the occurrence of phagocytosis.
    d. a and b.
    e. a and c.

36. (d,171)

36. A patient is diagnosed with lobar pneumonia. Which of the following exudates would be present in highest concentration?

    a. serous
    b. purulent
    c. hemorrhagic
    d. fibrinous

37. (c,171)

37. The cleanup of a lesion involving the dissolution of fibrin clots by fibrinolytic enzymes is:

    a. dissolution.
    b. reconstruction.
    c. debridement.
    d. none of the above.

38. (a,175)

38. A patient with scurvy generally expresses impaired healing due to a lack of:

    a. ascorbic acid.
    b. vitamin E.
    c. vitamin K.
    d. pyridoxine.

Matching

39. (e,166)	39. ___ interferon	a.	acute phase reactants
40. (c,166)	40. ___ tumor necrosis factor	b.	lysome-containing granulocytes
41. (g,166)	41. ___ interleukin-1	c.	produced in response to gram-negative sepsis
42. (a,169)	42. ___ plasma proteins	d.	differentiated macrophages
43. (d,170)	43. ___ epithelioid cells	e.	defends against viruses
44. (b,166)	44. ___ esinophils	f.	macrophage precursors
45. (f,164)	45. ___ monocytes	g.	produced in response to tissue injury

Short Answer

46. What two ways do mast cells use to activate the inflammatory response?

47. What are the four effects of activation of Hageman factor?

48. List the four types of exudate and give an example of each.

49. What are the two phases of resolution and repair?

50. Give three examples of dysfunctional wound healing.

Short Answers

46. 1. Degranulation
    2. Mediator synthesis (152)
47. 1. Activation of the clotting cascade through factor XI
    2. Generation of plasmin
    3. Activation of the kinin system
    4. Activation of C-1 in the complement cascade (160)
48. 1. Serous: a blister
    2. Fibrinous: lobar pneumonia
    3. Purulent or suppurative: abscess
    4. Hemorrhagic: laceration (171)
49. 1. Reconstructive phase
    2. Maturation phase (172)
50. 1. Prolonged healing
    2. Impaired collagen synthesis—keloid
    3. Impaired epithelialization
    4. Wound disruption—dehiscence
    5. Impaired contraction—contracture (175-176)

Hypersensitivities, Infection, and Immunodeficiencies

Name _____

True/False

1. (T,204)	1. T	F	Severe combined immune deficiency is a congenital immunodeficiency.
2. (T,207)	2. T	F	Deficient zinc intake can depress both T- and B-cell function.
3. (F,204)	3. T	F	Hypogammaglobulinemia is an acquired immunodeficiency.
4. (F,189)	4. T	F	Systemic lupus erythmatosis (SLE) is an alloimmune disease.
5. (T,191)	5. T	F	Humans harbor large numbers of beneficial microorganisms.
6. (T,191-192)	6. T	F	The first line of defense against pathogens is the skin and mucous membrane.
7. (F,196)	7. T	F	Viruses produce exotoxins.

Multiple Choice

8. (b,190)   8. A person with SLE is likely to have presence of:

    a.   anti-LE antibodies.
    b.   antinuclear antibodies.
    c.   antiherpes antibodies.
    d.   anti-CMV antibodies.

9. (d,181-183)   9. It is generally accepted that factors which contribute to hypersensitivity are:

    a.   genetic.
    b.   infectious.
    c.   environmental.
    d.   all of the above.

10. (c,181)   10. Hypersensitivity is best defined as:

    a.   a reduced immune response found in most pathological states.
    b.   a normal immune response to an infectious agent.
    c.   an excessive or inappropriate response of the immune system to a sensitizing antigen.
    d.   antigenic desensitization.

11. (a,182)

11. Seasonal allergic rhinitis, is expressed through:

    a. IgE-mediated reactions.
    b. tissue specific reactions.
    c. antigen-antibody complexes.
    d. type II hypersensitivity reactions.

12. (d,185)

12. Which of the following hypersensitivity reactions does not involve antibody?

    a. type I
    b. type II
    c. type III
    d. type IV

13. (d,181)

13. The class of antibody involved in type I hypersensitivity reactions is:

    a. IgG.
    b. IgM.
    c. IgA.
    d. IgE.

14. (c,181)

14. The most severe immediate hypersensitivity reaction is:

    a. urticaria.
    b. hives.
    c. anaphylaxis.
    d. ADCC.

15. (b,181)

15. Anaphylaxis:

    a. is always systemic.
    b. causes itching.
    c. causes hypertension.
    d. is not severe.

16. (d,186)

16. Graft rejection is caused by a type _____ reaction.

    a. I
    b. II
    c. III
    d. IV

17. (d,183-184)

17. Tests of IgE-mediated hypersensitivity include:

    a. radioimmunosorbent.
    b. radioallergosorbent.
    c. intradermal injection of allergen.
    d. all of the above.

18. (d,184)

18. Tissue-specific reactions are caused by each of the following mechanisms *except*:

    a. complement-mediated lysis.
    b. opsonization and phagocytosis.
    c. cellular malfunction.
    d. antigen-dependent cell-mediated cytotoxicity

19. (c,186)

19. Poison ivy is a form of:

   a.   anaphylaxis.
   b.   serum sickness.
   c.   type IV hypersensitivity.
   d.   lysosomal disease.

20. (d,186)

20. Tuberculin reaction is an example of type _____ hypersensitivity.

   a.   I
   b.   II
   c.   III
   d.   IV

21. (e,186)

21. George recently received a kidney transplant. Organ rejection occurred after two weeks. The primary mechanism for the rejection is:

   a.   immune response against recipient HLA antigens.
   b.   immune response against donor HLA antigens.
   c.   type IV hypersensitivity.
   d.   a and b.
   e.   b and c.

22. (a,189)

22. Autoimmunity may be caused by:

   a.   genetic predisposition.
   b.   anaphylaxis.
   c.   alloimmunity.
   d.   increased tolerance.

23. (b,189)

23. When the maternal immune system becomes sensitized against antigens expressed by the fetus, _____ disease is a result.

   a.   autoimmune
   b.   alloimmmune
   c.   homoimmune
   d.   alleimmune

24. (a,189)

24. Systemic lupus erythematosis is an example of:

   a.   autoimmunity
   b.   alloimmunity
   c.   homoimmunity
   d.   alleimmunity

25. (d,190)

25. The serial or simultaneous presence of at least _____ of the 11 signs or symptoms of systemic lupus erythematosus (SLE) are sufficient for the diagnosis of SLE.

   a.   11
   b.   9
   c.   10
   d.   4

26. (d,191)

26. The only disease that has been eradicated by vaccination is:

    a.   cholera.
    b.   malaria.
    c.   plague.
    d.   smallpox.

27. (c,191)

27. Which relationship benefits the organism but causes no harm to the host?

    a.   symbiosis
    b.   mutualism
    c.   commensalism
    d.   pathogenicity

28. (a,195)

28. Pathogens can defend themselves from an immune response by:

    a.   producing capsules.
    b.   phagocytosis.
    c.   commensalism.
    d.   developing antibodies.

29. (a,196)

29. Endotoxins are produced by:

    a.   gram negative bacteria.
    b.   gram positive bacteria.
    c.   gram negative fungi.
    d.   gram positive fungi.

30. (c,198)

30. Viruses:

    a.   contain no DNA or RNA.
    b.   are capable of independent reproduction.
    c.   produce proteins for replication.
    d.   are easily killed by antimicrobials.

31. (d,199)

31. Fungi causing deep or systemic infection:

    a.   die with antibiotic therapy.
    b.   are extremely rare.
    c.   never occur with other infections.
    d.   can be life threatening.

32. (a,200)

32. The hallmark of most infectious diseases is:

    a.   fever.
    b.   jaundice.
    c.   vomiting.
    d.   pain.

33. (b,202)

33. Most viral vaccines contain:

    a.   active viruses.
    b.   attenuated viruses.
    c.   killed viruses.
    d.   viral toxins.

34. (c,202)   34. Most bacterial vaccines contain:

        a.   active bacteria.
        b.   attenuated bacteria.
        c.   killed bacteria.
        d.   bacterial toxins.

35. (d,202-203)   35. Bacteria become resistant to antibiotics by:

        a.   proliferation.
        b.   attenuation.
        c.   specialization.
        d.   mutation.

36. (a,204)   36. If an immune deficiency has a clear genetic cause, it is called a _____ immunodeficiency.

        a.   primary
        b.   secondary
        c.   mild
        d.   severe

37. (b,204-205)   37. _____ is a condition in which immunoglobins are extremely low or absent.

        a.   Hypogammaglobinemia
        b.   Agammaglobinemia
        c.   Hypergammaglobinemia
        d.   None of the above

38. (b,206)   38. Congenital thymic aplasia is characteristic of:

        a.   Bruton disease.
        b.   DiGeorge syndrome.
        c.   ADA disease.
        d.   PNP syndrome.

39. (b,207)   39. AIDS is an example of a _____ immune disease.

        a.   primary
        b.   secondary
        c.   congenital
        d.   severe combined

40. (e,207)   40. More than half of all AIDS cases are in:

        a.   North America.
        b.   South America.
        c.   Europe.
        d.   Asia.
        e.   Africa.

41. (d,204)   41. Which of the following is a true statement?

        a.   Primary immune deficiency is caused by viral infections.
        b.   Secondary immune deficiency is caused by a genetic predisposition.
        c.   Both primary and secondary immune deficiencies result from cancer or viral infection.
        d.   Secondary immune deficiency may result from normal physiologic changes.

42. (d,208)   42. Acquired immune deficiency syndrome is transmitted via:

  a. sex with an infected person.
  b. contaminated blood transfusion.
  c. intrauterine transfer from mother to fetus.
  d. all of the above.

43. (b,210)   43. Which of the following is a characteristic of the human immunodeficiency virus (HIV), which causes AIDS?

  a. It only infects T-helper cells.
  b. The virus is a retrovirus.
  c. Infections usually do not require a cell receptor.
  d. Following viral infection, cell death is immediate.

44. (e,210-212)   44. Clinical manifestations of AIDS include:

  a. dementia.
  b. opportunistic infections.
  c. recurrent fevers.
  d. dysfunctional motor coordination.
  e. all of the above.

45. (b,216)   45. A common symptom of individuals with immunodeficiency is:

  a. anemia.
  b. recurrent infections.
  c. hypersensitivity.
  d. autoantibody production.

Matching

46. (b,193)   46. ___ infectivity   a. ability to induce an immune response

47. (e,193)   47. ___ pathogenicity   b. ability to invade and multiply in a host

48. (d,193)   48. ___ virulence   c. virulence of a pathogen

49. (a,193)   49. ___ antigenicity   d. potency of a pathogen

50. (c,193)   50. ___ toxigenicity   e. ability to produce disease

Short Answer

51. AIDS causes a striking decrease in _____ cells.

52. For every diagnosed AIDS case, how many others are estimated to be HIV-infected?

53. The replacement therapy for deficient antibody production is _____.

54. List three typical allergins.

55. List five symptoms of systemic lupus erythematosus.

Short Answers

51. CD4 or T-helper (212)
52. 100 (214)
53. Gamma globulin (217)
54. Pollens, molds, fungi, animals, foods, cigarette smoke, components of house dust (187)
55. Malar rash, discoid rash, photosensitivity, oral or nasopharyngeal ulcers, nonerosive arthritis of at least two joints, serositis, renal disorder, neurologic disorders, hematologic disorders, immunologic disorders, presence of antinuclear antibodies (190)

Stress and Disease

Name _____

True/False

1. (F,222)

1. T F "Fight or flight" is expressed in the exhaustion stage in the general adaptation syndrome (GAS).

2. (T,224)

2. T F Homeostasis may be defined as a dynamic steady state representing the net effect of all the turnover reactions.

3. (F,224)

3. T F Cortisol, an important compound in the body's response to stress, circulates in the plasma entirely free or unbound.

4. (T,225)

4. T F Cortisol enhances the elevation of serum glucose.

5. (T,225)

5. T F Catecholamines increase lipolysis.

6. (F,226)

6. T F Stress generally causes an increase in testosterone secretion.

7. (T,227)

7. T F There is evidence suggesting that the immune and neuroendocrine systems are connected through hormones common to both systems.

8. (F,227)

8. T F Stress has no effect on asthma.

9. (F,227)

9. T F The stress response is not influenced by the immune system.

10. (T,229)

10. T F There are direct effects of CNS and ANS neuropeptides on immune cells.

Multiple Choice

11. (c,222)

11. Exhaustion occurs if stress continues and _____ is not sucessful.

    a. fight or flight
    b. alarm
    c. adaptation
    d. arousal

12. (a,222)

12. The body's counteracting a physiological stress is referred to as:

    a. adaptation.
    b. general stress syndrome.
    c. DiGeorge syndrome.
    d. fight or flight.

13. (a,222)

13. The general adaptation syndrome (GAS) identified by Hans Selye, can be divided into stages and includes all of the following *except*:

   a. induction.
   b. exhaustion.
   c. alarm.
   d. resistance or adaptation.

14. (b,222)

14. Selye reported several structural changes in rats exposed to repeated stressors. These included:

   a. hypertrophy of the thymus gland.
   b. ulceration in the gastrointestinal system.
   c. atrophy of the cortex in the adrenal gland.
   d. fight or flight response.

15. (e,222)

15. Components of physiologic stress include:

   a. the body's adaptational response to the stressor.
   b. the stressor itself.
   c. the physical or chemical disturbance produced by the stressor.
   d. b and c.
   e. a, b, and c.

16. (a,224)

16. _____ best describes homeostasis.
   a. Dynamic steady state
   b. Steady state
   c. Constant composition
   d. Turnover composition

17. (c,224)

17. CRF stimulates the _____ gland to release a variety of hormones.

   a. adrenal
   b. hypothalamus
   c. pituitary
   d. thalamus

18. (d,224)

18. The process of synthesis and breakdown of all bodily substances is known as:

   a. anabolism.
   b. catabolism.
   c. dynamism.
   d. turnover.

19. (c,224)

19. _____ activates both alpha and beta receptors.

   a. cortisol.
   b. prolactin.
   c. epinephrine.
   d. somatotropin.

20. (d,225)

20. Catecholamines cause:

   a. smooth muscle contraction.
   b. increased glycogenolysis.
   c. smooth muscle relaxation.
   d. all of the above.

21. (a,227)

21. The initiation of the stress response is caused mainly by the nervous and endocrine systems but also involves:

    a. all of the following.
    b. the adrenal gland.
    c. the immune system.
    d. the pituitary gland.
    e. the sympathetic nervous system.

22. (c,224)

22. Stress induces sympathetic stimulation of the adrenal medulla. This causes the secretion of catecholamines, which include:

    a. epinephrine and aldosterone.
    b. norepinephrine and cortisol.
    c. epinephrine and norepinephrine.
    d. cortisol and aldosterone.

23. (b,224)

23. Stress-induced stimulation of the cortex of the adrenal gland causes it to secrete:

    a. estrogen.
    b. cortisol.
    c. parathyroid hormone.
    d. adrenocorticotropin hormone.

24. (a,224)

24. _____ from the hypothalamus stimulates the release of ACTH from the anterior pituitary.

    a. CRF
    b. Pituitary releasing factor
    c. ADH
    d. Oxytocin

25. (a,225)

25. Cortisol causes blood glucose levels to:

    a. increase.
    b. decrease.
    c. not change.

26. (b,224)

26. Stress-induced catecholamine release from the adrenal medulla may result in:

    a. decreased blood flow to the brain and skin.
    b. peripheral vasoconstriction.
    c. increased glycogen synthesis in the liver.
    d. decreased muscle contraction due to an energy depletion.

27. (a,224-225)

27. Stress may result in:

    a. increased action by catecholamines.
    b. decreased blood glucose.
    c. systemic decrease in protein synthesis.
    d. increased peripheral uptake and utilization of glucose.

28. (b,226)

28. Cortisol does all of the following *except*:

    a. delays healing.
    b. decreases protein absorption.
    c. increases lipolysis in the extremities.
    d. promotes gastric secretion.

29. (a,226)

29. Beta endorphins appear to regulate:

a. ACTH.
b. prolactin.
c. sex hormones.
d. insulin

30. (e,229)

30. Psychosocial distress may predict which health outcome(s)?

a. psychologic
b. social
c. physical
d. a and b
e. a, b, and c

31. (d,223)

31. Coping is best defined as the process of:

a. adjusting to disease.
b. preventing psychological distress.
c. mediating anger.
d. managing stressful challenges.

Matching

32. (b,223)

32. ___ norepinephrine   a. released from anterior pituitary

33. (e,223)

33. ___ epinephrine   b. released from nerve endings

34. (a,223)

34. ___ ADH   c. released from posterior pituitary

35. (c,223)

35. ___ ACTH   d. released from adrenal cortex

36. (d,223)

36. ___ cortisol   e. relased from adrenal medulla

Short Answer

37. Why do men have a higher morbidity than women following injury?

38. List three hormones that function in the stress response.

39. What are the three stages of Selye's GAS?

40. List three immune changes that occur with aging.

Short Answers

37. Testosterone exhibits immunosuppressive activity after injury. Estrogen enhances the immune response. (226)
38. Epinepherine, norepinepherine, cortisol, beta-endorphins, growth hormone, prolactin, testosterone, estrogen (226)
39. Alarm, resistance or adaptation, exhaustion (222)
40. Alterations in the excitability of structures of the limbic system and hypothalamus
    Rise of the blood concentration of catecholamines, ADH, ACTH, and cortisol
    Decrease of testosterone, thyroxine, and others
    Alterations in opioid peptides
    Hypercoagulation of blood
    Imunodepression
    Alterations in lipoproteins
    Free radical damage to cells

CHAPTER

9

Biology of Cancer

Name _____

True/False

1. (T,236)   1. T F   Anaplasia is the loss of cellular differentiation and organization.

2. (F,236)   2. T F   Autonomy refers to a cancer cell's dependence on normal cellular control mechanisms.

3. (T,237)   3. T F   As malignant cells grow, they often become less clearly differentiated.

4. (T,238)   4. T F   Some tumors closely mimic normal tissue.

5. (F,238)   5. T F   Cancer cells secrete fibrinogen-activating factor.

6. (T,237)   6. T F   Grade IV tumors are poorly differentiated.

7. (T,243)   7. T F   A person may be genetically predisposed to cancer.

8. (F,252)   8. T F   There is current evidence which associates obesity with cancer formation in men.

9. (T,254)   9. T F   Increased number of sexual partners has been shown to be related to the incidence of cervical cancer.

10. (F,255)   10. T F   There appears to be no relation between the incidence of melanoma and age at the time of exposure to excessive UV radiation.

Multiple Choice

11. (d,235)   11. A tumor may result when social control genes become:

    a.   active.
    b.   inactive.
    c.   overactive.
    d.   b and c.
    e.   a, b, and c.

12. (a,235)   12. A social control gene may lose its normal function because of:

    a.   mutation.
    b.   age.
    c.   hormonal changes.
    d.   none of the above.

13. (b,236) | 13. The process by which a cell acquires specific new observable characteristics is:

a. commitment.
b. differentiation.
c. commutation.
d. consanguination.

14. (a,236) | 14. Undifferentiated cells are:

a. stem cells.
b. all tumor cells.
c. committed cells.
d. T cells.
e. B cells.

15. (a,236) | 15. Tumors are classified on the basis of all of the following *except*:

a. DNA content.
b. benign versus malignant.
c. degree of differentiation.
d. anatomic site and function.
e. tissue of origin.

16. (c,238) | 16. _____ refers to preinvasive epithelial tumors of glandular or squamous cell origin.

a. Tumor in differentiation
b. Premetastatic
c. Cancer in situ
d. Cancer beyond (meta) situ

17. (b,235-236) | 17. An oncogene is best defined as:

a. a normal gene.
b. an altered gene.
c. an inactive gene
d. a tumor-supressor gene.

18. (b,239) | 18. Which of the following represents the correct nomenclature for benign and malignant tumors of adipose tissue, respectively?

a. liposarcoma, lipoma
b. lipoma, liposarcoma
c. adisarcoma, adipoma
d. adipoma, adisarcoma

19. (a,238) | 19. All of the following represent general characteristics of cancerous cells *except*:

a. decreased nuclear size.
b. local increase in cell number.
c. abnormal cellular arrangement.
d. variation in cell shape and size.

20. (d,241)

20. A patient is diagnosed as having a tumor in the pituitary gland. Which of the following would most likely show elevated levels?

a. calcium
b. serotonin
c. gastrin
d. prolactin

21. (c,238)

21. Tumors of the central nervous system are called:

a. carcinomas.
b. lymphomas.
c. gliomas.
d. leukemias.

22. (d,239)

22. All of the following characteristics are standard features of cancerous tissues *except*:

a. local increase in cell number.
b. loss of normal cell arrangement.
c. variation in cell size.
d. secretion of hormones in a regulated fashion.

23. (d,240)

23. Narrow channels between cells used for intercellular communication are called:

a. desmosomes.
b. hemidesmosomes.
c. homodesmosomes.
d. gap junctions.

24. (d,240)

24. Tumor cell markers can be used:

a. to screen individuals for cancer.
b. to diagnose tumor type.
c. to follow clinical course of tumor.
d. all of the above.

25. (b,241)

25. Normal cells, when grown in culture, follow social rules and respect each other's space; tumor cells do not respect each other's space and pile on top of each other. Tumor cells do not demonstrate:

a. contact inhibition.
b. density-dependent inhibition.
c. mutual respect.
d. any of the above.

26. (e,243-247)

26. The cause of cancer can be:

a. genetic.
b. environmental.
c. occupational.
d. a and b.
e. all of the above.

27. (b,236)   27. The process by which a normal cell becomes a cancer cell is:

   a. anaplasia.
   b. transformation.
   c. grading.
   d. differentiation.

28. (d,249)   28. The two-stage mechanism for the development of cancer includes:

   a. initiation and proliferation.
   b. proliferation and reduction.
   c. proliferation and promotion.
   d. initiation and promotion.

29. (c,249)   29. Which of the following is the main requirement for the initiation-promotion-projection theory of carcinogenesis?

   a. The promoting agent must act first.
   b. The initiating agent alone causes cancer formation.
   c. The initiating agent must act first, followed by action of the promoting agent.
   d. The initiating and promoting agents act independently.

30. (e,249)   30. Which of the following may be considered initiators and/or promoters?

   a. personal behaviors
   b. drugs
   c. hormones
   d. a and b
   e. a, b, and c

31. (b,251)   31. Smoking is associated with cancers of all of the following *except*:

   a. lung.
   b. skin.
   c. bladder.
   d. kidney.
   e. pancreas.

32. (a,254)   32. Which of the following compounds has been shown to increase the risk of cancer when used in combination with smoking?

   a. alcohol
   b. steroids
   c. antihistamines
   d. antidepressants

33. (d,254-255)   33. Which of the following viruses may be involved in increasing the incidence of cervical cancer?

   a. herpes simplex virus type 2
   b. rubella virus
   c. human papillomavirus
   d. a and c
   e. a and b

34. Which of the following is a true statement?

    a. Pregnancy appears to increase the risk of endometrial cancer.
    b. Early onset of menstruation may decrease the risk of breast cancer.
    c. Pregnancy at an early age may increase the risk of breast cancer.
    d. Pregnancy may protect against cancer of the ovaries.

35. Indoor pollution is considered worse than outdoor pollution because of:

    a. cigarette smoke.
    b. radon gas.
    c. benzene.
    d. a and b.
    e. none of the above.

36. Which of the following is the main assumption in the immune surveillance theory of carcinogenesis?

    a. Cancer cells do not express "nonself" antigens.
    b. In the nonpathological state, tumor "nonself" antigens are accepted.
    c. Tumor-associated antigens are similar to those found on normal, nontransformed cells.
    d. Cancer cells express "nonself" antigens, which, in the normal individual, are recognized and rejected.

37. Tumors may "escape" immunologic rejection by:

    a. production of blocking antibodies.
    b. secretion of immunosuppressive substances and antigenic modulation.
    c. selective stimulation of suppressor cells.
    d. a and c.
    e. a, b, and c.

Matching

38. ___   carcinoma   a. cancer of bone marrow

39. ___   lymphoma   .b. cancer of epithelial tissue

40. ___   leukemia   c. cancer of lymphatic tissue

41. ___   glioma   d. cancer of central nervous system

Short Answer

42. List three cellular characteristics of cancerous tissue.

43. List three tumor cell markers.

44. List two proposed mechanisms by which malignant cells become autonomous.

45. List three ways tumors escape immunologic rejection.

Short Answers

42. Local increase in cell number
    Loss of normal cell arrangement
    Variation in cell shape and size
    Increase in nuclear size and density of staining
    Increase in mitiotic activity
    Abnormal mitosis and chromosomes (238)
43. Hormones, enzymes, genes, antigens, antibodies (240)
44. Manufacture by transformed cells of their own growth factors
    Reduction in the amount of growth factor necessary for cell division
    Defects of the growth factor receptor on the plasma membrane
    Alteration of the receptor signal pathway for second messengers (242)
45. Antigenic modulation
    Secretion of immunosuppressive substances
    Escape and sneaking through
    Blocking factor
    Immunostimulation
    TSA-reactive suppressor T-lymphocytes (262)

Tumor Spread and Treatment

Name _____

True/False

1. (T,270)

1. T   F   Direct mechanical pressure may be a part of the mechanism of local tumor spreading.

2. (T,270)

2. T   F   Tumors may spread into surrounding areas by first digesting away the normal tissue.

3. (T,271)

3. T   F   Often primary tumors are not diagnosed until a metastatic secondary tumor has been discovered.

4. (F,273)

4. T   F   All tumor cells that are released into the blood eventually find a compatible tissue to multiply in and give rise to a tumor.

5. (F,273)

5. T   F   The metastatic potential of many common carcinomas is related to the size of the tumors.

6. (T,277)

6. T   F   Erythropoietin is an effective treatment for anemia for people with cancers.

7. (T,278)

7. T   F   Curative resections of tumors are performed if distant metastasis is not evident.

Multiple Choice

8. (d,271)

8. Tumors may spread throughout the body and can take several forms *except*:

   a.   direct invasion of contiguous organs.
   b.   metastasis via veins or lymphatics.
   c.   metastasis via implantation.
   d.   metastasis by encystment.

9. (e,271)

9. Spreading of a tumor can occur by:

   a.   direct extension.
   b.   metastasis via lymph.
   c.   metastasis via blood.
   d.   b and c.
   e.   all of the above.

10. (a,271)   10. Metastasis can be defined as the process where tumors spread from primary to distant sites. Which of the following shows a correct sequence in the process of metastasis?

    a. local extension, penetration into blood/lymph, transport
    b. transport, vascularization, adherence of tumor cells
    c. vascularization, invasion into lymph and vascular systems, transport
    d. vascularization, local extension, transport

11. (b,270)   11. Tumors are known to secrete _____, which is a lytic enzyme.

    a. lanolinase
    b. collagenase
    c. endorphin
    d. trypsin

12. (d,273)   12. Preferential metastatic growth in certain organs is called organ:

    a. intravasation.
    b. extravasation.
    c. diapedesis.
    d. tropism.

13. (c,270)   13. Tumor cells may secrete _____ in order to promote their own movement.

    a. monokines
    b. cytokines
    c. autocrine motility factors
    d. none of the above

14. (e,273)   14. Which of the following may not be the fate of a tumor cell that becomes lodged in a lymph node?

    a. death because of the local inflammation it causes
    b. death because of an incompatible local environment
    c. sustained dormancy
    d. detachment from the nodes into the efferent lymphatics
    e. detachment from the nodes into the afferent lymphatics

15. (a,275)   15. The syndrome of cachexia includes all of the following signs and symptoms *except*:

    a. normal carbohydrate metabolism.
    b. early satiety.
    c. weight loss.
    d. anorexia.

16. (a,274-276)   16. All of the following are clinical manifestations of cancer *except*:

    a. weight gain.
    b. anemia.
    c. fatigue.
    d. cachexia.

17. (b,275)   17. Basal metabolic rates of people with cancer are usually _____ than normal.

    a. lower
    b. higher
    c. fluctuating more

18. (c,276)

18. Which of the following is not a possible cause of anemia in people with cancers?

    a.   chronic bleeding
    b.   iron deficiency
    c.   magnesium deficiency
    d.   medical therapies

19. (d,278)

19. Biological response modifiers are:

    a.   chemotherapy agents.
    b.   antimetabolites.
    c.   nitroureas.
    d.   immunotherapies.

20. (c,277)

20. All of the following represent goals of radiation therapy *except*:

    a.   to eradicate cancer.
    b.   to avoid damage to normal structures.
    c.   to replace chemotherapy.
    d.   to prevent excessive toxicity.

21. (d,277)

21. To be curative, chemotherapy must eradicate:

    a.   all of the tumor cells.
    b.   all of the cycling cells.
    c.   all of the cells not cycling.
    d.   enough so that the body's own defense system can clean up the remaining cells.

22. (a,274)

22. The most frequently reported symptom of cancer and cancer treatment is:

    a.   fatigue.
    b.   anorexia.
    c.   pain.
    d.   weight loss.

Matching

23. (d,277)   23. ____ chemotherapy   a. actual tumor removal

24. (b,277)   24. ____ radiation   b. direct ionization

25. (a,277)   25. ____ surgery   c. eliminates cancer cells, spares normal tissue

26. (c,278)   26. ____ immunotherapy   d. targets replication processes

Short Answer

27. What is the most significant cause of complications and death in people with cancer?

28. List two causes of leukopenia in people with cancer.

29. What are the three steps in the hypothesis of tumor invasion?

30. What is the most common route for distant metastasis?

Short Answers

27. Infection (277)
28. Direct tumor invasion of bone marrow
    Chamotherapy
    Radiotherapy (277)
29. Attachment, dissolution, locomotion (272)
30. Through the lymphatics (272)

Cancer in Children

Name _____

True/False

1. (T,283)

2. (F,284-286)

3. (T,287)

4. (F,286)

5. (F,286)

1. T F Childhood cancer is the second leading cause of death in children.

2. T F Childhood cancer is seen much more frequently in black children.

3. T F Diethylstilbestrol, DES, acts as a transplacental chemical carcinogen.

4. T F Early warning signs of cancer in adults are also reliable indicators in children.

5. T F Incidence of cancer in children increases with age.

Multiple Choice

6. (c,284)

6. Most childhood cancers originate from the:

    a. placenta.
    b. environment.
    c. mesodermal germ layer.
    d. neural tube.

7. (d,284)

7. Embryonic tumors are:

    a. nonmalignant.
    b. frequently seen in adults.
    c. composed of mature, differentiated cells.
    d. usually manifested by age 5.

8. (a,284)

8. The most common malignancy in children is:

    a. leukemia.
    b. neuroblastoma.
    c. Wilms tumor.
    d. retinoblastoma.

9. (b,286)

9. The incidence by gender for childhood cancer is:

    a. equal.
    b. higher in boys.
    c. higher in girls.
    d. unknown.

Matching: Processes associated with childhood cancer

10. (c,287)	10. ___ chromosome alteration	a. agammaglobulinemia
11. (e,287)	11. ___ chromosome instability	b. cryptorchidism
12. (d,287)	12. ___ heredity syndrome	c. Down syndrome
13. (a,287)	13. ___ immunodeficiency disorder	d. neurofibromatosis
14. (b,287)	14. ___ congenital malformation	e. Fanconi anemia

Short Answer

15. A 9-month-old monozygotic twin is diagnosed with leukemia. What is the probability that the other twin will develop it?

16. What is the probability if the twins are 3 years old?

17. What is the probability if the twins are 10 years old?

18. Hepatitis C infection in childhood puts an individual at great risk for developing what cancer as an adult?

19. What parental behavior increases a child's risk for all childhood cancers?

20. What percentage of children with cancer will survive?

Short Answers

15. Nearly 100% (287)
16. 15% (287)
17. It is equal to that of the general population. (287)
18. Liver cancer (288)
19. Cigarette smoking (289)
20. 60% (289)

CHAPTER

12

Structure and Function of the Neurologic System

Name _____

True/False

1. (F,295)	1. T F Chemical synapses between neurons can send messages in both directions.
2. (F,292)	2. T F The central nervous system is composed of the brain, spinal cord, cranial nerves, and spinal nerves.
3. (T,307)	3. T F Cerebrospinal fluid exerts pressure within the brain and spinal cord.
4. (F,307)	4. T F Approximately 300 cc of cerebrospinal fluid are produced each day.
5. (F,307)	5. T F The spinal cord has no direct blood supply and receives its nutrition exclusively from cerebrospinal fluid.
6. (F,312)	6. T F The bloodbrain barrier is composed of the three meninges covering the brain cells.
7. (F,317)	7. T F The fight or flight response is primarily mediated by the parasympathetic nervous system.
8. (T,318)	8. T F The craniosacral system is the parasympathetic branch of the autonomic nervous system.
9. (F,318)	9. T F Beta adrenergic receptors are part of the parasympathetic system.
10. (F,320)	10. T F Cholinergic effects on heart muscles increase heart rates, increase contractility, and increase propagation velocity of impulses through ventricles.
11. (T,318)	11. T F The parasympathetic nervous system functions to conserve and restore energy.
12. (T,321)	12. T F A major function of sympathetic nervous system cells is regulation of blood vessel tone.
13. (F,307)	13. T F Oxygen is the primary regulator of blood flow within the CNS.
14. (F,308)	14. T F Cerebral venous drainage parallels the arterial supply.

Multiple Choice

15. (a,292)   15. _____ pathways carry sensory information.

   a.   Ascending
   b.   Descending
   c.   Galea
   d.   Meningeal

16. (a,292)   16. The axon leaves the cell body at a single:

   a.   axon hillock.
   b.   axonal nissl body.
   c.   dendritic hillock.
   d.   synaptic hillock.

17. (b,293)   17. Which of the following transmit a nerve impulse at the highest rate?

   a.   large nonmyelinated axons
   b.   large myelinated axons
   c.   small nonmyelinated axons
   d.   small myelinated axons

18. (d,312)   18. A cell that apparently is part of the blood-brain barrier is a:

   a.   neurolemmacyte.
   b.   Schwann cell.
   c.   oligodendrocyte.
   d.   astrocyte.

19. (d,294)   19. Which of the following is not a neuroglial cell?

   a.   astrocyte
   b.   oligodendrocyte
   c.   ependymal cell
   d.   neuron

20. (d,295)   20. Regeneration of an injured nerve depends on:

   a.   location of injury.
   b.   type of injury.
   c.   inflammatory response.
   d.   all of the above.

21. (a,295)   21. Neurotransmitters interact with the _____ membrane by binding to a _____.

   a.   postsynaptic, receptor
   b.   presynaptic, receptor
   c.   axonal, receptor
   d.   axonal, lipid

22. (e,296)   22. Examples of a neurotransmitter might include:

   a.   histamine.
   b.   dopamine.
   c.   glutamic acid.
   d.   endorphins.
   e.   all of the above.

23. (a,295)

23. A neurotransmitter may:

a.   prevent a postsynaptic cell from sending, or cause it to send, an action potential.
b.   prevent a presynaptic neuron from sending, or cause it to send, an action potential.
c.   cause a postsynaptic cell to send an action potential only.
d.   cause a presynaptic cell to send an action potential only.

24. (b,295)

24. If a neuron's membrane potential is held close to the threshold potential by EPSPs, the neuron is said to be:

a.   hyperpolarized.
b.   facilitated.
c.   integrated.
d.   all of the above.

25. (b,297)

25. The _____ is a large network of neurons within the brain stem that is essential for maintaining wakefulness.

a.   corpora quadragemina
b.   reticular activating system
c.   cerebellum
d.   hypothalamus

26. (a,301)

26. Vital reflex centers for respiration and cardiovascular function are primarily located in the:

a.   brain stem.
b.   hypothalamus.
c.   thalamus.
d.   cerebral cortex.

27. (c,299)

27. Elaboration of thought and goal-oriented behavior are functions of the _____ area of the brain.

a.   thalamus
b.   limbic system
c.   prefrontal
d.   occipital lobe

28. (a,299)

28. Damage to the _____ would result in the impairment of fine repetitive motor movements.

a.   extrapyramidal system
b.   prefrontal area
c.   Wernicke area
d.   temporal lobe
e.   Broca area

29. (b,299)

29. At the inferior margin of the precentral gyrus is the region responsible for motor aspects of speech; this area is termed:

a.   Wernicke area
b.   Broca area
c.   Midas area
d.   none of the above

30. (b,300)   30. The _____ is a _____ fiber tract that connects the two cerebral hemispheres.

a. peduncle, projection
b. corpus callosum, transverse
c. corpus callosum, projection
d. corpus callosum, association

31. (d,297)   31. The convolutions on the surface of the cerebrum are called:

a. sulci.
b. fissures.
c. rectular formations.
d. gyri.

32. (e,300)   32. The _____ has two main functions, maintenance of homeostasis and instinctive behavioral control.

a. thalamus
b. medulla
c. cerebellum
d. pons
e. hypothalamus

33. (b,301)   33. The ability of the eyes to track moving objects through a visual field is primarily a function of the:

a. inferior colliculi.
b. superior colliculi.
c. corpora quadrigemini.
d. all of the above

34. (e,300)   34. Functions of the hypothalamus include:

a. temperature regulation.
b. awakeness.
c. autonomic nervous system activity.
d. a and c.
e. a, b, and c.

35. (d,301)   35. The _____ controls reflex activities concerned with heart rate, blood pressure, respirations, sneezing, swallowing, and coughing.

a. pons
b. midbrain
c. cerebellum
d. medulla oblongata
e. none of the above

36. (d,301)   36. A patient with altered respiratory patterns may have a lesion of the:

a. cerebrum.
b. cerebellum.
c. midbrain.
d. hindbrain.

37. (b,304)	37. Characteristics of upper motor neurons include:

    a.   directly influencing muscles.
    b.   influencing and modifying spinal reflex arcs.
    c.   their cell bodies being located in the gray matter of the spinal cord.
    d.   their dendritic processes extending out of the CNS.

38. (a,306)	38. The _____ is the membrane that surrounds the brain stem and separates the cerebellum from the cerebrum.

    a.   tentorium cerebelli
    b.   falx cerebri
    c.   arachnoid membrane
    d.   falx cerebelli

39. (a,306)	39. The outermost membrane surrounding the brain is the:

    a.   dura mater.
    b.   arachnoid.
    c.   meninges.
    d.   faux cerebri.

40. (b,307)	40. _____ produce cerebrospinal fluid.

    a.   Arachnoid villi
    b.   Choroid plexuses
    c.   Ependymal cells
    d.   Ventricles

41. (e,307)	41. CSF circulates within the:

    a.   ventricles.
    b.   subarachnoid space.
    c.   foramen of Munro.
    d.   a and b.
    e.   all of the above.

42. (b,307)	42. The brain receives approximately _____ of the cardiac output.

    a.   80%
    b.   20%
    c.   40%
    d.   10%

43. (c,308)	43. The _____ ensures collateral blood flow from blood vessels supplying the brain.

    a.   carotid arteries
    b.   basal artery
    c.   circle of Willis
    d.   vertebral arteries

44. (d,308)	44. The circle of Willis is formed by several arteries, one of which is the:

    a.   vertebral artery.
    b.   midcerebral artery.
    c.   basilar artery.
    d.   anterior communicating artery.

Matching

45. (e,315)	45. ___ glossopharyngeal	a. tested by ability of eye muscles to follow moving objects
46. (d,315)	46. ___ oculomotor	
		b. has both motor and sensory functions to face, mouth, nose, and eyes
47. (a,315)	47. ___ trochlear	
48. (f,315)	48. ___ abducens	c. carries motor functions to tongue and sensory impulses from tongue to brain
49. (b,315)	49. ___ trigeminal	
		d. controls size, shape, and equality of pupils and medial rectus eye muscles
		e. causes motor functions to pharynx and salivary glands and sensory functions from pharynx and tongue
		f. carries motor actions to lateral rectus muscle and proprioceptor fibers from same muscle to brain

Short Answer

50. What does the somatic nervous system regulate?

51. List the four basic structural types of neurons.

52. List the three functional types of neurons.

53. What are the three major divisions of the brain?

54. Where does the subdural space lie?

55. What are the two arterial systems that supply blood to the brain?

Short Answers

50. It regulates voluntary motor control in skeletal muscles. (292)
51. Unipolar, pseudounipolar, bipolar, and multipolar (293)
52. Sensory, associational, and motor (293)
53. Forebrain, midbrain, hindbrain (297)
54. It lies between the dura and arachnoid membrane (306)
55. The internal carotid arteries and the vertebral arteries (307)

Pain, Temperature, Sleep, and Sensory Function

Name _____

True/False

1. (F,326)	1. T F	Acute anxiety is not usually associated with acute pain.
2. (F,326)	2. T F	Psychogenic pain is pain with a known physical cause.
3. (F,326)	3. T F	Hopelessness frequently accompanies acute pain experiences.
4. (T,326)	4. T F	A person's pain threshold does not vary significantly over time.
5. (T,326)	5. T F	Acute pain is a protective mechanism.
6. (F,326)	6. T F	The nociceptors are at the ends of the large myelinated efferent neurons.
7. (T,326)	7. T F	The sensitivity to pain differs in different body areas.
8. (T,328)	8. T F	Large A fibers transmit sharp, localized pain sensations.
9. (T,329)	9. T F	Endorphins inhibit transmission of pain impulses.
10. (F,328)	10. T F	The "gate theory" of pain control states that a "closed gate" increases pain perception.
11. (T,329)	11. T F	All endorphins act by attaching to opiate receptors on the plasma membranes of afferent neurons.
12. (F,330)	12. T F	Persistent chronic pain produces a physiologic response similar to that of acute pain.
13. (T,331)	13. T F	Neuralgias are painful conditions that result from an infection or disease that damages a peripheral nerve.
14. (T,330)	14. T F	Temperature regulation is mediated hormonally by the hypothalamus.
15. (F,331)	15. T F	The adrenal medulla is not a target tissue for thyroxine.
16. (T,332)	16. T F	Fever is not the result of a failure of normal thermoregulatory mechanisms.

Multiple Choice

17. (a,326)

17. _____ is the duration of time or the intensity of pain that a person will endure before outwardly responding to it.

    a.   Pain tolerance
    b.   Pain perception
    c.   Pain threshold
    d.   None of the above

18. (d,326)

18. The portions of the nervous system responsible for the sensation and perception of pain are all of the following *except*:

    a.   afferent pathways.
    b.   central nervous system.
    c.   efferent pathways.
    d.   autonomic motor pathways.

19. (c,326)

19. The efferent pathways are composed of fibers connecting the reticular formation, the midbrain, and the:

    a.   red nucleus.
    b.   basal ganglia.
    c.   substantia gelatinosa.
    d.   all of the above.

20. (d,326)

20. Nociceptors are located in:

    a.   tissues.
    b.   spinal cord.
    c.   efferent pathways.
    d.   hypthalamus.

21. (b,328)

21. The _____ tract is responsible for carrying information to the brain concerning dull and burning pain.

    a.   neospinothalamic
    b.   paleospinothalamic
    c.   archeospinothalamic
    d.   a and b
    e.   a, b, and c

22. (a,326)

22. Chronic pain is pain that has lasted longer than:

    a.   6 months.
    b.   1 year.
    c.   18 months.
    d.   2 years.

23. (d,329)

23. _____ are a family of neuropeptides that inhibit the transmission of pain impulses in the spinal cord and brain.

    a.   Endorphins
    b.   Enkaphalins
    c.   Dynorphins
    d.   All of the above

24. (e,330)   24. _____ cause(s) an increase in the levels of circulating endorphins.

      a. Acupuncture
      b. Excessive physical exertion
      c. Stress
      d. Intercourse
      e. All of the above

25. (b,330)   25. All of the following are types of acute pain *except*:

      a. somatic.
      b. impulsive.
      c. visceral.
      d. referred.

26. (c,326)   26. _____ pain is a warning of actual or impending tissue injury.

      a. Chronic
      b. Psychogenic
      c. Acute
      d. Impulsive

27. (b,327)   27. Pain threshold in children is:

      a. higher than that of adults.
      b. lower than that of adults.
      c. the same as that of adults.
      d. not related to that of adults.

28. (c,331)   28. _____ is pain that an individual feels in an amputated limb after the stump has completely healed.

      a. Agnosia
      b. Hyperagnosia
      c. Phantom limb pain
      d. Paragnosia

29. (c,331)   29. One way that the hypothalamus functions in raising body temperature is by relaying information to the _____ to provoke heat conservation.

      a. cerebellar cortex
      b. insula
      c. cerebral cortex
      d. medulla oblongata

30. (a,331)   30. Why do infants have problems with thermoregulation?

      a. They cannot conserve heat.
      b. They do not shiver.
      c. They rarely sweat.
      b. They have decreased metabolic rates.

31. (a,331)   31. All of the following are mechanisms of heat loss *except*:

      a. peripheral vasoconstriction.
      b. radiation.
      c. conduction.
      d. convection.

32. (b,333)

32. Accidental hyperthermia that results in profuse sweating is:

    a.   heat cramps.
    b.   heat exhaustion.
    c.   heat stroke.
    d.   malignant hyperthermia.

33. (b,332)

33. _____ is a mechanism for preserving body temperature.

    a.   Involuntary vasodilation of peripheral blood vessels
    b.   Voluntary mechanism (e.g., movement, clothing)
    c.   Decreased muscle tone
    d.   Increased respiration

34. (b,332)

34. _____ are exogenous pyrogens.

    a.   Arginine vasopressins
    b.   Endotoxins
    c.   Alpha-melanocyte stimulating hormones
    d.   Corticotropin-releasing factors

35. (a,332)

35. For evaporation to function effectively in heat loss, _____ must be present.

    a.   moisture
    b.   fever
    c.   pyrogens
    d.   heat stroke
    e.   trauma

36. (c,333)

36. Seizures in children below age five are frequently the result of:

    a.   meningitis.
    b.   epilepsy.
    c.   fever.
    d.   morbidity.

37. (c,333)

37. The form of accidental hyperthermia a person will not get when working in the heat is:

    a.   heat exhaustion.
    b.   heatstroke.
    c.   malignant hyperthermia.
    d.   heat cramps.

38. (b,334)

38. In acute hypothermia, _____ shunts blood away from the colder skin to the body core in an effort to decrease heat loss.

    a.   peripheral vasodilation
    b.   peripheral vasoconstriction
    c.   visceral vasoconstriction
    d.   all of the above

39. (c,335)

39. _____ is known as paradoxical sleep.

    a.   Non-REM sleep
    b.   Light sleep
    c.   REM sleep
    d.   Delta wave sleep

40. (a,335-336)

40. _____ are characterized by sudden apparent arousals in which a child expresses intense fear or other emotion.

   a. Night terrors
   b. Nightmares
   c. Somnambulisms
   d. None of the above

41. (c,335)

41. Loss of temperature control occurs in:

   a. non-REM sleep
   b. light sleep
   c. REM sleep
   d. delta wave sleep

42. (d,340)

42. Viral conjunctivitis is caused by:

   a. secondary bacterial infections.
   b. cytomegalovirus.
   c. herpes virus.
   d. adenovirus.

43. (a,326)

43. Pain tolerance may be decreased by all of the following *except*:

   a. rest.
   b. anger.
   c. fatigue.
   d. apprehension.

44. (c,330)

44. Referred pain from the liver may be felt in the:

   a. flank.
   b. left arm.
   c. right shoulder.
   d. buttocks.

45. (b,335)

45. A disorder that results in excessive somnolence is:

   a. insomnia.
   b. obstructive sleep apnea syndrome.
   c. somnambulism.
   d. jet-lag syndrome.

46. (c,330)

46. Regulation of body temperature primarily occurs in which part of the brain?

   a. cerebrum
   b. brain stem
   c. hypothalamus
   d. pituitary gland

47. (c,332)

47. Release (increase) of epinephrine increases body temperature by:

   a. increasing shivering.
   b. increasing muscle tone.
   c. increasing heat production.
   d. decreasing basal metabolic rate.

48. (b,332)   48. Heat loss from the body via convection occurs by:

    a.   emanations of electromagnetic waves.
    b.   transfer of heat through currents of liquids or gas.
    c.   dilations of blood vessels bringing blood to skin surfaces.
    d.   direct heat loss from molecule to molecule transfer.

49. (b,333)   49. Characteristics of heat stroke include:

    a.   core temperatures usually reaching about 101° F.
    b.   degeneration of the CNS.
    c.   rapidly decreasing core temperature as heat loss from the evaporation of sweat ceases.
    d.   being caused by calcium release or decreased clacium uptake.

50. (c,334)   50. Theraputic hypothermia is seen in:

    a.   malnutrition.
    b.   hypotheyroidism.
    c.   reimplantation surgery.
    d.   Parkinson's disease.

51. (d,335)   51. Rapid eye movement (REM) sleep occurs about every:

    a.   15 minutes.
    b.   30 minutes.
    c.   60 minutes.
    d.   90 minutes.

52. (d,335)   52. Which is not a special sense?

    a.   taste
    b.   hearing
    c.   smell
    d.   pain

Matching

53. (f,338)   53. ____   scotoma   a. loss of ability to smell

54. (g,337)   54. ____   nystagmus   b. perversion of sense of taste

55. (d,337)   55. ____   amblyopia   c. smelling nonexistent odors

56. (e,340)   56. ____   organ of Corti   d. reduced vision in one eye

57. (a,343)   57. ____   anosmia   e. contains receptor cells for hearing

58. (b,344)   58. ____   parageusia   f. defect in central field of vision

                                                      g. involuntary movements of eyeballs

Short Anwer

59. Name the three systems that interact to produce pain.

60. Define perceptual dominance.

61. What neurons transmit diffuse burning or aching sensations?

62. List four mechanisms of heat loss.

63. At what temperature does death result?

64. What are the four major classification of sleep disorders?

65. What are the three types of refraction?

Short Anwers

59. Sensory/discriminative, motivational/affective, and cognitive/evaluative (326)
60. Pain threshold is the lowest intensity at which a stimulus is perceived as pain. Intense pain at one location may increase the threshold in another location. This is perceputal dominance. (326)
61. Small unmyelinated C neurons (328)
62. Radiation, conduction, convention, vasodilation, decreased muscle tone, evaporation, increased respiration, voluntary measures, and adaptation to warmer climates. (331)
63. 43° C or 109.4° F (333)
64. Disorders of initiating sleep; disorders of excessive somnolence; disorders of the sleep-wake cycle; and dysfunctions of sleep, sleep stages, or partial arousals (335)
65. Myopia, hyperopia, and astigmatism (338)

Concepts of Neurologic Dysfunction

Name _____

True/False

1. (F, 351)

2. (T, 351)

3. (T, 351)

4. (F, 355)

5. (T, 355)

6. (T, 356)

7. (F, 362)

8. (F, 365)

9. (T, 369)

10. (F, 370)

1. T F   Consciousness and content of thought comprise arousal.

2. T F   Disorders outside the brain, but within the cranial vault, can cause altered arousal.

3. T F   Level of consciousness is the most critical index of nervous system function.

4. T F   Yawning, vomiting, and hiccups are simple relex-like motor responses.

5. T F   When evaluationg pupillary response in unconscious individuals, one must take into account the drugs the individual has received.

6. T F   A convulsion is one form of seizure.

7. T F   Aphasia is the impairment of comprehension or production of language.

8. T F   All dementias are secondary to other events.

9. T F   Hydrocephalus can develop in adults.

10. T F   Hypertonia can be caused by cerebellar damage.

Multiple Choice

11. (c,351)

12. (e,351)

11. Arousal is mediated by the:

    a. cerebral cortex.
    b. medulla oblongata.
    c. reticular activating system.
    d. cingulate gyrus.

12. The reticular activating system controls:

    a. arousal.
    b. content of thought.
    c. affective states.
    d. a and b.
    e. all of the above.

13. (c,351)   13. Possible causes of an altered level of arousal may include any of the following *except*:

a. structural.
b. metabolic.
c. sociologic.
d. psychogenic.

14. (e,355)   14. Dilated fixed pupils can be caused by:

a. large doses of atropine.
b. severe ischemia.
c. hypoxia.
d. b and c.
e. a, b, and c.

15. (d,355)   15. Vomiting is particularly associated with CNS injuries that involve all of the following *except*:

a. vestibular nuclei.
b. floor of the fourth ventricle.
c. brain stem compression.
d. frontal lobe.

16. (c,355)   16. Irreversible coma is:

a. brain death.
b. supratentorial brain death.
c. cerebral death.
d. brain stem death.

17. (b,356)   17. A sudden, explosive, disorderly discharge of cerebral neurons is:

a. reflex.
b. seizure.
c. epilepsy.
d. none of the above.

18. (a,359)   18. Etiologic factors in seizures generally include all of the following *except*:

a. diplopia.
b. cerebral lesions.
c. biochemical disorders.
d. cerebral trauma.
e. metabolic defects.

19. (e,359)   19. Seizures are classified by:

a. site of origin.
b. EEG correlates.
c. response to therapy.
d. clinical manifestations.
e. all of the above.

20. (e,359)

20. Seizures can be diagnosed using:

    a. computed tomography scan (CT).
    b. cerebrospinal fluid analysis.
    c. laboratory tests.
    d. a and b.
    e. all of the above.

21. (d,359)

21. A peculiar sensation that immediately precedes a seizure is called:

    a. prodroma.
    b. agnosia.
    c. spasm.
    d. aura.

22. (b,350)

22. Neural networks basic to cognitive functions include.

    a. attentional networks.
    b. memory and language networks.
    c. affective systems.
    d. a and b.
    e. a, b, and c.

23. (c,362)

23. _____ is a defect in recognition, a failure to recognize the form and nature of objects.

    a. Aphasia
    b. Dysphasia
    c. Agnosia
    d. None of the above

24. (b,362)

24. _____ is the loss of production or comprehension of language.

    a. Dyspnea
    b. Aphasia
    c. Apnea
    d. Agnosia

25. (c,366)

25. Cortical dementia is manifested by all of the following *except*:

    a. apraxia.
    b. loss of recent memory.
    c. depression.
    d. loss of remote memory.

26. (a,366)

26. Normal intracranial pressure in mm of Hg is:

    a. 5-15.
    b. 7-20.
    c. 12-14.
    d. 80-120.

27. (b,369)

27. _____ is the straight downward shift of the diencephalon through the tentorial notch.

    a. Uncal herniation
    b. Central herniation
    c. Cingulate herniation
    d. Infratentorial herniation

28. (b,368)   28. Cerebral edema is an increase in the fluid content of:

    a. brain ventricles.
    b. brain tissue.
    c. CNS neurons.
    d. none of the above.

29. (d,368)   29. The clinically most important cerebral edema is:

    a. ischemic.
    b. interstitial.
    c. metabolic.
    d. vasogenic.

30. (b,369)   30. _____ edema is most often seen with noncommunicating hydrocephalus.

    a. Metabolic
    b. Interstitial
    c. Vasogenic
    d. Ischemic

31. (c,367)   31. A compensatory alteration in the diameter of cerebral blood vessels in response to increased intracranial pressure is called:

    a. vasoconstriction.
    b. vasodilation.
    c. autoregulation.
    d. amyotrophy.

32. (d,353)   32. The least altered level of consciousness is _____; the most altered is _____.

    a. disorientation; stupor
    b. disorientation; coma
    c. confusion; stupor
    d. confusion; deep coma

33. (a,373)   33. _____ refers to paralysis of the lower extremities.

    a. Paraplegia
    b. Quadriplegia
    c. Infraparaplegia
    d. Supraparaplegia
    e. None of the above

34. (b,373)   34. _____dyskinesia is the involuntary movements of the face, trunk, and extremities.

    a. Paroxysmal
    b. Tardive
    c. Hyper-
    d. Cardrive

35. (c,373)   35. _____ is excessive movement.

    a. Tachykinesia
    b. Akinesia
    c. Hyperkinesia
    d. Dyskinesia

36. (a,378-379)   36. A _____ is a senile gait.

    a. basal ganglion gait
    b. cerebellar gait
    c. supraganglion gait
    d. scissors gait

Mr. Walt Elliot is admitted to the intensive care unit with a severe closed head injury.

37. (a,368)   37. This diagnosis puts Mr. Elliot at risk for:

    a. cerebral edema.
    b. metabolic coma.
    c. dysphagia.
    d. echolalia.

38. (b,358)   38. The nurse notes Mr. Elliot with all four extremities in rigid extension and with forearm hyper pronation and legs with plantar extension. This is known as:

    a. decorticate posturing.
    b. decerebrate posturing.
    c. caloric posturing.
    d. excitation posturing.

39. (a,366)   39. When an intraventricular catheter is inserted, the intracranial pressure is 24 mm Hg. This reading is:

    a. higher than normal.
    b. lower than normal.
    c. normal.
    d. borderline.

40. (c,367)   40. Mr. Elliot's condition is deteriorating. His pupils are small and sluggish, his pulse pressure is widening, and the pulse is bradycardic. These clinical findings are evidence of what stage of intracranial hypertension?

    a. stage 1
    b. stage 2
    c. stage 3
    d. stage 4

41. (b,367)   41. Increased intracranial pressure in one cranial compartment is evenly distributed throughout the other cranial compartments.

    a. true
    b. false

42. (b,355-356)   42. When thought content and arousal level are intact but a patient cannot communicate, the patient has:

    a. agnosia.
    b. locked-in syndrome.
    c. dysphagia.
    d. cerebellar motor syndrome.

43. (c,360)

43. Ms. Smith has a seizure which starts with her fingers and progressively spreads up the arm and extends to the leg. This is known as:

    a. myoclonic seizure.
    b. tonic-clonic seizure.
    c. Jacksonian seizure.
    d. atonic seizure.

44. (b,362)

44. Since his cerebral vascular accident, Mr. Thomas has been denying his left hemiplegia. This is a form of:

    a. amusia.
    b. agnosia.
    c. alexia.
    d. agraphia.

45. (d,362)

45. Mr. Thomas also has dysphasia. Most language disorders are caused by occlusion of the:

    a. anterior communicating artery.
    b. posterior communicating artery.
    c. circle of Willis.
    d. middle cerebral artery.

46. (e,362)

46. Agnosia can be:

    a. tactile.
    b. visual.
    c. auditory.
    d. a and b.
    e. all of the above.

47. (d,374)

47. Spinal shock is characterized by all of the following *except*:

    a. flaccid paralysis.
    b. vasodilation.
    c. disturbed bladder function.
    d. intact bowel function.

Matching

48. (d,364)

48. ____ expressive dysphasia

49. (c,364)

49. ____ receptive dysphasia

50. (b,377)

50. ____ decrease in voluntary movement

51. (a,373)

51. ____ abnormal involuntary movement

a. dyskinesia

b. akinesia

c. Wernicke dysphagia

d. Broca dysphagia

e. flaccidity

Short Answer

52. List the five categories that are critical to evaluating altered levels of arousal.

53. List one example of hemispheric breathing patterns and one example of brain stem breathing patterns.

54. What are the two extrapyramidal motor syndromes?

55. What is the difference between paresis and paralysis?

Short Answers

52. Level of consciousness, pattern of breathing, size and reactivity of pupils, eye position and reflexive responses, and skeletal muscle motor responses (351)
53. Hemispheric: normal, posthyperventilation apnea, Cheyne-Stokes
Brain stem: central neurogenic hyperventilation, apneusis, cluster breathing, ataxic breathing, agonal respiration (353)
54. The basal ganglia motor syndromes and the cerebellar motor syndromes (379)
55. Paresis is partial or incomplete loss of muscle power. Paralysis is complete loss of motor function. (373)

Alterations of Neurologic Function

Name _____

True/False

1. (F,392)

1. T F Autonomic dysreflexia is most likely to occur before spinal shock is resolved.

2. (T,392)

2. T F Because spinal cord swelling increases the degree of dysfunction, it is difficult to distinguish between permanent and temporary loss of function until the swelling is resolved.

3. (T,396)

3. T F In quadriplegia the level of injury is in the cervical vertebrae.

4. (T,399)

4. T F Strokes tend to run in families.

5. (F,400)

5. T F Abnormal heart structure does not put a person at risk for embolic strokes.

6. (T,402)

6. T F In cases of subarachnoid hemorrhage the intercranial pressure rises dramatically.

7. (F,415)

7. T F CNS tumors are the most common type of tumors in children.

8. (F,409)

8. T F Parkinson disease shows a very clear inheritance pattern.

9. (T,410)

9. T F Huntington disease is inherited as an autosomal dominant trait with high penetrance.

10. (F,411)

10. T F The peripheral nervous system is the main location of lesions in multiple sclerosis.

11. (F,411)

11. T F Multiple sclerosis demonstrates a well-defined inheritance pattern.

12. (T,392)

12. T F Spinal shock results in a temporary loss of reflex function below the spinal cord lesion.

Multiple Choice

13. (a,388)

13. The most severe diffuse brain injury caused by rotational acceleration is most likely to be located:

   a. more peripheral to the brain stem.
   b. in the medial portion of the brain stem.
   c. throughout the brain stem.
   d. distal to the brain stem.

14. (e,398)

14. If a person has diffuse brain injury, he or she is most likely to show which of the following clinical manifestations?

    a. physical consequences
    b. cognitive deficits
    c. behavioral manifestations
    d. a and b
    e. a, b, and c

15. (d,390)

15. _____ are most at risk of spinal cord injury from minor trauma.

    a. Infants
    b. Men
    c. Women
    d. The elderly
    e. a and d

16. (c,390)

16. Which of the following is the least likely site of vertebral injury (cervical, C; thoracic, T; lumbar, L)?

    a. C1 to C2
    b. C4 to C7
    c. T4 to T5
    d. T12 to L2

17. (c,392)

17. Indications that spinal shock is terminating include all of the following *except*:

    a. reappearance of reflex activity.
    b. reflex emptying of the bladder.
    c. loss of spasticity.
    d. hyperreflexia.

18. (b,392)

18. The initial clinical manifestations associated with acute spinal cord injury are all of the following *except*:

    a. loss of sensation below the level of the injury.
    b. loss of autonomic reflexes above the injury.
    c. loss of voluntary control below the injury.
    d. loss of spinal reflexes below the injury.

19. (c,392)

19. If a person has had a spinal cord injury above T6 about three weeks previous to experiencing paroxysmal hypertension and has piloerection and sweating above the spinal cord lesion, she is likely to be experiencing:

    a. craniosacral dysreflexia.
    b. parasympathetic dysreflexia.
    c. autonomic hyperreflexia.
    d. healing of the spinal cord lesion.

20. (e,399)

20. All of the following are risk factors for thrombotic strokes *except*:

    a. hypothyroidism.
    b. sickle cell disease.
    c. polycythemia vera.
    d. use of oral contraceptives.
    e. fat emboli.

21. (e,400) | 21. Conditions associated with the onset of embolic stroke include:

    a. endocarditis.
    b. atrial fibrillation.
    c. myocardial infarction.
    d. valvular prostheses.
    e. all of the above.

22. (a,399) | 22. Of the following, who are at highest risk for a cerebrovascular accident?

    a. blacks over 65 years of age
    b. whites over 65 years of age
    c. blacks under 65 years of age
    d. whites umder 65 years of age

23. (b,415) | 23. Most intracranial tumors in children are located:

    a. supratentorially.
    b. infratentorially.
    c. laterally.
    d. posteriolaterally.

24. (c,416) | 24. _____ are the most common primary CNS tumors.

    a. Microgliomas
    b. Neuroblastomas
    c. Astrocytomas
    d. Neuromas

25. (d,418) | 25. Meningiomas usually arise from:

    a. dura mater.
    b. arachnoid cells.
    c. pia mater.
    d. a and b.
    e. all of the above.

26. (d,403) | 26. Meningitis may be caused by:

    a. bacteria.
    b. viruses.
    c. fungi.
    d. all of the above.

27. (b,411) | 27. The central component of the pathogenic model of multiple sclerosis is:

    a. demyelination of nerve fibers in the PNS.
    b. demyelination of nerve fibers in the CNS.
    c. the development of neurofibril tangles in the CNS.
    d. the development of neurofibril tangles in the PNS.

28. (a,387) | 28. Mr. Sam Jackson, 25, was in an automobile accident. At impact, Mr. Jackson's forehead struck the windshield. In this situation, the coup injury would occur in the:

    a. frontal region.
    b. temporal region.
    c. parietal region.
    d. occipital region.

29. (d,387)   29. Mr. Jackson's contracoup injury would occur in the:

  a.   frontal region
  b.   temporal region
  c.   parietal region
  d.   occipital region

Bill Henderson, 17, is brought to the emergency department for treatment of injuries received in a motor vehicle accident. A spinal cord injury is suspected.

30. (d,390)   30. As a nurse, you know the spinal cord is more easily injured in the areas of the spinal column where the cord occupies most of the vertebral canal. The two regions where this is the case are the:

  a.   cervical and thoracic regions
  b.   thoracic and lumbar regions
  c.   lumbar and sacral regions
  d.   cervical and lumbar regions

31. (c,392)   31. It is determined that Bill has an injury of the cervical cord. You know cord swelling in this region may be life-threatening because:

  a.   increased intracranial pressure may occur
  b.   reflexes will be disrupted
  c.   diaphragm function may be impaired
  d.   bladder emptying will not occur

32. (b,392)   32. Bill's body temperature fluctuates markedly. The most accurate explanation of this phenomenon is that:

  a.   Bill has probably developed pneumonia
  b.   Bill's sympathetic nervous system has been damaged and thermal control disturbed
  c.   urinary tract infections are common in persons with Bill's injury
  d.   Bill has septicemia from an unknown source

33. (c,392)   33. Bill's condition stabilizes after one week. Suddenly he develops a blood pressure of 250/120, a severe headache, blurred vision, and bradycardia. Bill is diagnosed as:

  a.   experiencing acute anxiety regarding his upcoming surgery
  b.   developing extreme spinal shock
  c.   developing autonomic hyperreflexia
  d.   experiencing parasympathetic areflexia

34. (c,400)   34. Mr. Armstrong, 72, demonstrates left-sided weakness of upper and lower extremities. The symptoms dissapper in 24 hours. He most likely experienced a:

  a.   stroke-in-evolution.
  b.   lacunar.
  c.   transient ischemic attack.
  d.   cerebral hemorrhage.

35. (e,400)   35. Lacunar strokes are associated with:
  a.   an embolus.
  b.   a thrombus.
  c.   a hemorrhage.
  d.   an aneurysm.
  e.   hypertension.

36. (c,400)

36. A major contributing process in CVA is the development of atheromatous plaques in cerebral circulation. These most commonly form:

   a. in the larger veins.
   b. near capillary sphincters.
   c. in cerebral arteries.
   d. in the venous sinuses.

37. (d,409)

37. Bob Jones, 61, develops tremors and muscle stiffness. Following a neurological work-up, he is diagnosed as having Parkinson disease. This is a degenerative disorder of the:

   a. hypothalamus.
   b. adrenals.
   c. pituitary.
   d. basal ganglia.

38. (d,409)

38. In teaching Mr. Jones about his disease, you explain that it causes his body to lack the inhibitory neurotransmitter called:

   a. antidiuretic hormone.
   b. adrenalin.
   c. acetylcholine.
   d. dopamine.

39. (a,411)

39. Susan Taylor, 23, begins having problems with tiredness, weakness, and visual changes. Her diagnosis is multiple sclerosis (MS). The best description of MS is:

   a. central nervous system demyelination, possibly due to an immunogenetic-viral cause.
   b. inadequate supply of acetylcholine at the neuromuscular junction due to an autoimmune disorder.
   c. depletion of dopamine in the central nervous system due to viral, vascular, or metabolic factors.
   d. a degenerative disorder of lower and upper motor neurons due to viral-immune factors.

Matching

40. (b,385)

40. ___ one of the most common traumatic brain injuries

41. (e,386)

41. ___ bleeding into the brain tissue

42. (c,385)

42. ___ accumulation of blood, usually arterial, above dura mater but beneath the skull

43. (d,385-386)

43. ___ collection of blood, usually between dura mater and the arachnoid membrane

44. (a,388)

44. ___ results from a shaking effect to the brain

a. diffuse axonal injury
b. concussion
c. extradural hematoma
d. subdural hematoma
e. intracerebral hematoma venous,

Short Answer

45. List three causes of CNS alterations.

46. In classic cerebral concussion, how long is consciousness lost?

47. List four symptoms of postconcussive syndrome.

48. How long does spinal shock last?

49. What signs and symptoms are seen in a Hunt-Hess grade V subarachnoid hemorrhage?

50. What are four causes of meningitis?

Short Answers

45. Traumatic injury, vascular disorder, tumor growth, infectious and inflammatory processes, metabolic derangements, and degenerative processes (384)
46. Up to six hours (389)
47. Headache, nervousness or anxiety, irritability, insomnia, depression, inability to concentrate, forgetfulness, and fatigability (389)
48. 7 to 20 days (392)
49. Deep coma, decerebrate posturing, signs of brain stem functioning (403)
50. Bacteria, viruses, fungi, parasites, and toxins (403)

Alterations of Neurologic Function in Children

Name _____

True/False

1. (T,426)

   1. T F   Many reflex patterns mediated by brain stem and spinal cord mechanisms are present and should disappear at predictable times.

2. (F,428)

   2. T F   Meningoceles occur at a greater frequency in the lumbar spine area.

3. (T,430)

   3. T F   Spina bifida occulta occurs in 10% to 25% of infants.

4. (F,426)

   4. T F   By three months of age, the anterior fontanelle is closed in the normal developmental process.

5. (F,431)

   5. T F   Congenital hydrocephalus is a leading cause of mental retardation.

6. (F,434)

   6. T F   Incidence of epilepsy varies greatly with age.

7. (F,433)

   7. T F   Tay-Sachs disease is an autosomal dominant disease.

8. (T,434)

   8. T F   Pica occurs most often in two- to three-year-olds.

9. (T,434)

   9. T F   The occurrence of Reye syndrome has decreased with public awareness of the association between the ingestion of aspirin during illness and the subsequent development of Reye syndrome.

10. (F,439)

   10. T F   A neuroblastoma (an embryonal tumor) arises from the same cells that would normally develop into the parasympathetic nervous system.

Multiple Choice

11. (d,428)

   11. The first reflex of infancy to disappear is:

      a. stepping.
      b. rooting.
      c. palmar grasp.
      d. Moro's reflex.

12. (e,430)

12. Causes of microcephaly include:

    a. defects in brain development.
    b. intrauterine infections.
    c. perinatal and postnatal disorders.
    d. both a and c.
    e. a, b, and c.

13. (c,426)

13. Which of the following is a true statement:

    a. Head circumference increases until puberty.
    b. All normal reflexes are present at birth.
    c. Neonatal reflexes disappear in a predictable order.
    d. a and b.
    e. all of the above.

14. (b,428)

14. _____ defects of neural tube closure are most common.

    a. Anterior
    b. Posterior
    c. Lateral
    d. Superior
    e. Inferior

15. (c,428)

15. _____ is an anterior midline defect of neural tube closure.

    a. Anencephaly
    b. Myelodysplasia
    c. Cyclopia
    d. Hydrocephaly

16. (a,428)

16. _____ refers to a herniation or protrusion of brain and meninges through a defect in the skull.

    a. Encephalocele
    b. Meningocele
    c. Arachnoidocele
    d. Ancephalocele

17. (a,428-429)

17. Defects of the neural tube closure include all of the following *except*:

    a. congenital hydrocephalus.
    b. anencephaly.
    c. meningocele.
    d. encephalocele.
    e. myelomeningocele.

18. (b,430)

18. Which of the following is a valid characteristic of spina bifida?

    a. easily visible pathological state
    b. abnormal growth of hair along the spine
    c. condition occurring in less than 5% of all infants
    d. b and c
    e. a, b, and c

19. (a,430-431)
19. An infant is diagnosed with hydrocephalus. Which of the following characteristics would you expect to see?

    a.   enlarged ventricles
    b.   normal cerebrospinal fluid production and/or reabsorption
    c.   dilation of the cerebral aqueduct
    d.   decreased head circumference

20. (c, 432)
20. The most common type of cerebral palsy is:
    a.   mixed.
    b.   dyskinetic.
    c.   spastic.
    d.   ataxic.

21. (c,432-433)
21. Which of the following represent inherited metabolic disorders of the CNS?

    a.   Tay-Sachs, phenylketonuria, acrania
    b.   acrania, galactosemia, Tay-Sachs
    c.   Tay-Sachs, phenylketonuria, galactosemia
    d.   Tay-Sachs, phenylketonuria, craniosynostosis

22. (d,432)
22. Urine screens on newborns are performed to detect:

    a.   epilepsy.
    b.   Tay-Sachs disease.
    c.   pica.
    d.   PKU.

23. (b,436)
23. A child is brought to the emergency room. He is demonstrating the following clinical manifestations: tissue ischemia, anemia, and an apparent decrease in normal growth rate. Which of the following poisons to the CNS would most likely be the cause?

    a.   ethyl alcohol
    b.   lead
    c.   mercury
    d.   carbon monoxide
    e.   tranquilizers

24. (a,435)
24. The most common cause of bacterial meningitis in the U.S. is:

    a.   *Haemophilus influenzae.*
    b.   *Neisseria meningitidis.*
    c.   *Streptococcus pneumoniae.*
    d.   viruses.

25. (d,435)
25. Viral meningitis is:

    a.   always sudden in onset.
    b.   not seen secondary to other infections.
    c.   effectively treated with antibiotics.
    d.   aseptic.

26. (b,437)
26. The most common location of brain tumors in children is:

    a.   always above the cerebellum.
    b.   posterior fossa.
    c.   in the cerebrum.
    d.   in the ventricular lining.

27. (d, 429)

27. _____ is a hernial protrusion of a saclike cyst (containing meninges, spinal fluid, and a portion of the spinal cord with its nerves) through a defect in the posterior arch of a vertebra.

     a.   Encephalocele
     b.   Meningocele
     c.   Spina bifida occulta
     d.   Myelomeningocele

28. (e, 430)

28. _____ may indicate an underlying condition of spina bifida.

     a.   Abnormal growth of hair along the spine
     b.   A midline dimple posterior to the vertebral column
     c.   A cutaneous angioma
     d.   A subcutaneous mass
     e.   All of the above

29. (a,430)

29. Which of the following is (are) characterized by a premature closure of one or more of the cranial sutures?

     a.   craniosynostosis
     b.   craniosuture sclerosis
     c.   microcephaly
     d.   acrania
     e.   all of the above

30. (b,430)

30. True microcephaly can be caused by an _____ gene.

     a.   autosomal dominant
     b.   autosomal recessive
     c.   X-linked recessive
     d.   X-linked dominant

31. (c,437)

31. The most common site of HIV infection in children is:

     a.   the lungs.
     b.   the gastrointestinal tract.
     c.   the central nervous system.
     d.   the skin.

Matching

32. (b,432)   32. ___   inborn error of metabolism   a.   gestational brain injury

33. (c,434)   33. ___   encephalopathy   b.   PKU

34. (a,432)   34. ___   cerebral palsy   c.   Reye's syndrome

35. (d,439)   35. ___   sympathetic nervous system tumor   d.   neuroblastoma

36. (e,440)   36. ___   autosomal dominant tumor   e.   retinoblastoma

Short Answer

37. The posterior fontanelle closes by _____ months; the anterior, by _____ months.

38. During infancy, what is the fastest growing part of the body?

39. Where are most vertebral malformations found?

40. List two types of cerebral palsy.

Short Answers

37. 2 to 3; 6 (426)
38. The head (428)
39. The lumbosacral region (430)
40. Spastic, dyskinetic, ataxic (432)

Mechanisms of Hormonal Regulation

Name _____

True/False

1. (T,453)

1. T F   The pituitary gland located in the bony sella turcica approximately doubles it weight during pregnancy.

2. (F,456)

2. T F   Osmoreceptors do not affect the release of antidiuretic hormone (ADH).

3. (F,456)

3. T F   At physiologic levels, ADH decreases the permeability of the distal renal tubules and collecting ducts.

4. (T,461)

4. T F   The brain does not require insulin for glucose uptake.

5. (F,461)

5. T F   Glucagon is synthesized by the beta cells of the pancreas.

6. (T,462)

6. T F   Somatostatin is produced by the pancreas.

7. (T,464)

7. T F   ACTH directly affects the regulation of melanin levels in the skin melanocytes.

Multiple Choice

8. (b,446)

8. All of the following are basic secretion patterns of hormones *except*:

   a. pulsatile.
   b. constant.
   c. diurnal.
   d. substrate level dependent.

9. (a,460)

9. _____ slow down the rate of secretion of parathyroid hormone.

   a. Increased serum calcium levels
   b. Decreased serum calcium levels
   c. Decreased levels of TSH
   d. Increased levels of TSH

10. (c,446)

10. Regulation of the release of epinephrine from the adrenal medulla is an example of _____ regulation.

   a. negative feedback
   b. positive feedback
   c. neural
   d. substrate level dependent

11. (e,446)   11. Regulators of endocrine gland secretion include:

    a. negative feedback.
    b. other hormones.
    c. neural control.
    d. a and b.
    e. all of the above.

12. (d,447)   12. Which of the following is a protein hormone?

    a. thyroxine (T_4)
    b. aldosterone
    c. follicle stimulating hormone (FSH)
    d. insulin

13. (a, 447)   13. Which of the following is a polypeptide?

    a. adrenocorticotropic hormone (ACTH)
    b. triiodothyronine (T_3)
    c. epinephrine
    d. growth hormone (GH)

14. (b,447)   14. Protein hormones are primarily transported in the bloodstream:

    a. bound to a lipid-soluble carrier.
    b. free in an unbound, water-soluble form.
    c. bound to a water-soluble binding protein.
    d. free because of their lipid-soluble chemistry.

15. (d,449)   15. When insulin binds its receptors on muscle cells, an increase in glucose uptake by the muscle cells is the result. This is an example of a _____ effect by a hormone.

    a. pharmacologic
    b. permissive
    c. synergistic
    d. direct

16. (c,449)   16. ADH was originally named vasopressin because of its _____ effects.

    a. physiologic
    b. permissive
    c. pharmacologic
    d. synergistic

17. (d,450)   17. Target cell hormone receptors may _____ in order to change the cell's sensitivities to a given hormone concentration.

    a. be increased in concentration
    b. be decreased in concentration
    c. be changed in their affinity for a hormone
    d. all of the above

18. (a,449)   18. Lipid soluble hormone receptors cross the plasma membrane by:

    a. diffusion.
    b. osmosis.
    c. active transport.
    d. phagocytosis.

19. (e,449)

19. Hormone-receptor binding initiates an increase in the intracellular level of the second messenger. Which of the following statements is accurate about hormone-receptor binding?

   a. Hormone binding is regulated by intracellular and extracellular mechanisms.
   b. Hormone binding to plasma membrane receptors causes the release of second messengers like c-AMP.
   c. Once stimulated, c-AMP catalyzes the breakdown of glycogen to glucose.
   d. a and c.
   e. a, b, and c.

20. (a,451)

20. Which of the following hormones acts on its target cell via a second messenger?

   a. gonadotropin-releasing hormone
   b. thyroxin
   c. estrogen
   d. testosterone
   e. aldosterone

21. (b,449)

21. Receptors for most water-soluble hormones are located _____ of their target cells.

   a. in the cytosol
   b. in the cell membrane
   c. in the lysosomes
   d. all of the above

22. (c,449)

22. Calcium within cells:

   a. is controlled by the calcium-negative feedback loop.
   b. is continuously synthesized and utilized as a first messenger.
   c. regulates receptor affinity and/or acts as a second messenger.
   d. binds and carries lipid soluble hormones in the bloodstream.

23. (e,456)

23. The portion of the pituitary that secretes oxytocin is the:

   a. posterior.
   b. neurohypophysis.
   c. anterior.
   d. adenohypophysis.
   e. a and b.

24. (b,455)

24. A prolactin-inhibiting factor's target tissue is the:

   a. hypothalamus.
   b. anterior pituitary.
   c. mammary glands.
   d. posterior pituitary.

25. (a,456)

25. Antidiuretic hormone is synthesized by the:

   a. hypothalamus.
   b. infundibular stem.
   c. anterior pituitary.
   d. posterior pituitary.

26. (d,456)

26. Oxytocin is synthesized in the:

   a. hypothalamus.
   b. paraventricular nuclei.
   c. supraoptic nuclei.
   d. all of the above.

27. (d,457)

27. _____ affect(s) the level of antidiuretic hormone.

   a. Plasma osmolality
   b. Hypertension
   c. Pain
   d. a and c
   e. all of the above

28. (a,456)

28. Antidiuretic hormone is important in:

   a. the body's water balance and urine concentration.
   b. maintaining electrolyte levels and concentrations.
   c. follicular maturation.
   d. regulation of metabolic processes.

29. (b,456)

29. The releasing hormones that are made in the hypothalamus travel to the anterior pituitary via the:

   a. vessels of the zona fasciculata.
   b. infundibular stem.
   c. hypophysial stalk.
   d. portal system of the hypophysial arteries.

30. (e, 459)

30. Thyroid hormone is produced in response to:
   a. circulating TSH levels.
   b. low serum iodine levels.
   c. some drugs.
   d. b and c.
   e. a, b, and c.

31. (c,463)

31. The most potent naturally occurring glucocorticoid is:

   a. aldosterone
   b. testosterone
   c. cortisol
   d. prolactin

32. (b,459)

32. TSH:

   a. decreases the release of thyroid hormone.
   b. increases iodine uptake and oxidation.
   c. decreases the secretion of prostaglandins.
   d. increases insulin levels.

33. (d,458,460)

33. _____ is (are) secreted by the thyroid gland.

   a. Calcitonin
   b. Parathyroid hormone
   c. Thyroxine
   d. a and c
   e. a, b, and c

34. (c,459)

34. Which of the following is not involved in the regulation of thyroid hormone levels?

    a.   thyroxine
    b.   hypothalamus
    c.   posterior pituitary
    d.   anterior pituitary

35. (d,458,460)

35. _____ is (are) involved in the regulation of serum calcium levels.

    a.   Parathyroid hormone
    b.   Thyroxine
    c.   Calcitonin
    d.   a and c
    e.   all of the above

36. (d,457)

36. Target cells of oxytocin are located in the:

    a.   proximal convoluted tubules of nephrons.
    b.   distal convoluted tubules of nephrons.
    c.   glomeruli of nephrons.
    d.   uterus.

37. (b,462)

37. Which of the following is *not* secreted by the adrenal cortex?

    a.   cortisol
    b.   catecholamines
    c.   androgens
    d.   estrogens

38. (d, 466)

38. Adrenal catecholamines promote:

    a.   ACTH release.
    b.   aldosterone secretion.
    c.   hypotension.
    d.   hyperglycemia.

39. (a,463)

39. Metabolically, glucocorticoids cause:

    a.   protein catabolism and liver gluconeogenesis.
    b.   fat storage and glucose utilization.
    c.   decreased blood glucose and fat mobilization.
    d.   fat, protein, and carbohydrate anabolism.

40. (c, 462)

40. The main site of aldosterone syntheses is the:

    a.   liver.
    b.   kidneys.
    c.   adrenal glands.
    d.   hypothalamus.

41. (b, 465)

41. High levels of aldosterone may result in:

    a.   hyponatremia.
    b.   alkalosis.
    c.   hyperkalemia.
    d.   acidosis.

42. (d,447) | 42. All of the following are steroids *except*:

a. cortisol.
b. aldosterone.
c. androgens.
d. catecholamines.

Matching

43. (e,462) | 43. ___ zona glomerulosa   a. glucagon

44. (d,462) | 44. ___ zona fasciculata   b. catecholamines

45. (g,462) | 45. ___ zona reticularis   c. pancreatic polypeptide

46. (b,462) | 46. ___ adrenal medulla   d. cortisol

47. (a,460) | 47. ___ alpha cells of pancreas   e. aldosterone

48. (f,460) | 48. ___ beta cells of pancreas   f. insulin

49. (h,460) | 49. ___ delta cells of pancreas   g. adrenal androgens

50. (c,460) | 50. ___ F cells of pancreas   h. somatostatin

Short Answer

51. What are the five general functions of the endocrine system?

52. What organ(s) excrete(s) hormones?

53. List three structural categories of hormones.

54. List two laboratory tests used to measure hormone levels.

55. What general endocrine changes occur with aging?

Short Answers

51. Differentiation of fetal reproductive and endrocrine systems
    Stimulation of sequential growth and development during childhood and adolescence
    Coordination of the male and female reproductive systems
    Maintenance of an optimal internal environment
    Initiation of emergency corrective and adaptive responses (445)
52. Kidneys and liver (446)
53. Proteins, glycoproteins, polypeptides, amines, steroids, fatty acids (447)
54. Radioimmunoassay, enzyme-linked immunosorbent assay, bioassay (466)
55. Atrophy and weight loss with vascular changes; decreased secretion and clearance of hormones; variable change in receptor binding and intracellular responses (467)

Alterations of Hormonal Regulation

Name _____

True/False

1. (T,471)	1. T	F	Autonomous hormone production occurs in ectopic nonendocrine tissues.
2. (F,473)	2. T	F	Diabetes insipidus is caused by insufficient secretion of insulin.
3. (T,475)	3. T	F	Giantism occurs prior to epiphyseal closure.
4. (T,472)	4. T	F	A person with SIADH usually craves fluids.
5. (F,473)	5. T	F	Low serum osmolality is seen in SIADH.
6. (T,474)	6. T	F	ACTH deficiency is potentially life-threatening.
7. (F,477)	7. T	F	The most common cause of thyrotoxicosis is Cushing's disease.
8. (T,478)	8. T	F	Thyrotoxic crisis is also known as thyroid storm.
9. (T,481)	9. T	F	Myxedema coma is seen in severe hypothyroidism.
10. (F,486)	10. T	F	Hyperclycemia occurs when 50% of the beta cells are destroyed in the pancreas.

Multiple Choice

11. (a,471)

11. General types of abnormal target cell responses include:

    a. receptor-associated disorders.
    b. intercellular disorders
    c. increased synthesis of second messengers.
    d. extracellular disorders.

12. (b,472)

12. The syndrome of inappropriate ADH secretion (SIADH) is characterized by:

    a. low levels of ADH.
    b. high levels of ADH.
    c. anterior pituitary damage.
    d. a and c.

13. (d,472)

13. A diagnosis of SIADH requires:

    a.   serum hypoosmolality.
    b.   serum hyponatremia.
    c.   improvement of hyponatremia with water restriction.
    d.   all of the above.

14. (a,473)

14. Diabetes insipidus is related to:

    a.   ADH hyposecretion.
    b.   ADH hypersecretion.
    c.   hypothalamic hyperactivity.
    d.   b and c.

15. (c,472-473)

15. The control system for ADH may be ineffective in:

    a.   SIADH.
    b.   diabetes insipidus.
    c.   a and b.
    d.   none of the above.

16. (a,472)

16. The most common cause of elevated levels of ADH secretion is:

    a.   ectopically produced ADH.
    b.   inflammation of the hypothalamus.
    c.   hypothalamic injury.
    d.   inflammation of the optic nerve.

17. (a,472)

17. A 54-year-old patient with oat-cell adenocarcinoma of the lung is evaluated for SIADH by the nurse. Which of the following would the nurse expect to find if the patient had SIADH?

    a.   hyponatremia and hypoosmolality
    b.   hyperkalemia and serum hypoosmolality
    c.   hyponatremia and urine hyperosmolality
    d.   hypokalemia and serum hyperosmolality

A 22-year-old is admitted to the intensive care unit with a closed head injury sustained in a motorcycle accident. Within 24 hours, the patient's urine output is 6-8 L/day and electrolytes are within normal limits.

18. (a,473)

18. The nurse draws a serum ADH level and conducts a water-deprivation test. With no intake for four hours, there is no change in the patient's polyuria. The serum ADH level is low. This is indicative of:

    a.   neurogenic diabetes insipidus.
    b.   SIADH.
    c.   diabetes mellitus.
    d.   osmotically induced diuresis.

19. (d,472-473)

19. Diabetes insipidus, diabetes mellitus, and SIADH all have which of the following signs?

    a.   polyuria
    b.   edema
    c.   vomiting and abdominal cramping
    d.   thirst

20. (b,473)   20. A side effect of some general anesthetic agents is _____ diabetes insipidus.

    a. neurogenic
    b. nephrogenic
    c. psychogenic
    d. none of the above

21. (a,473)   21. Damage to the renal tubules would possibly result in _____ diabetes insipidus.

    a. nephrogenic
    b. neurogenic
    c. psychogenic
    d. none of the above

22. (a,473)   22. Type of diabetes insipidus that is likely to be treatable with exogenous ADH is:

    a. neurogenic.
    b. psychogenic.
    c. nephrogenic.
    d. all of the above.

23. (a,475)   23. Hyperpituitarism is generally caused by:

    a. a pituitary adenoma.
    b. hypothalamic hyposecretion.
    c. hypothalamic inflammation.
    d. a neurohypophyseal tumor.

24. (d,473)   24. Secondary hypopituitarism results from dysfunction of the:

    a. anterior pituitary.
    b. posterior pituitary.
    c. pars intermedia.
    d. hypothalamus.

25. (b,475)   25. _____ are a likely neurologic dysfunction resulting from a pituitary adenoma.

    a. Comas
    b. Visual disturbances
    c. Confusional states
    d. Breathing abnormalities

26. (e,475)   26. _____ is (are) caused by hypersecretion of growth hormone.

    a. Cushing syndrome
    b. Acromegaly
    c. Giantism
    d. Dwarfism
    e. b and c

27. (a,477)   27. Graves disease is characterized by:

    a. hypersecretion of thyroid hormone.
    b. hyposecretion of thyroid hormone.
    c. hyposecretion of thyroid stimulating hormone.
    d. none of the above.

28. (c,478)

28. Julia, a 25-year-old female, is admitted to your unit with Graves disease. You would expect to see which of the following signs on admission?

    a.   weight gain to 155 pounds with height of 5 feet 8 inches
    b.   heart rate 90/minute; respiratory rate 16/minute
    c.   skin hot and moist; protrusion of eyeballs
    d.   constipation; normal menses

29. (a,477)

29. Julia's Graves disease is usually characterized by:

    a.   high levels of circulating thyroid-stimulating immunoglobulins.
    b.   stimulation by thyroid-stimulating hormone (TSH) and thyrotropin-releasing hormone (TRH).
    c.   low circulating levels of thyroid hormones.
    d.   stimulation of thyroid-binding globulin.

30. (b,477)

30. The level of T_3 in Graves disease is usually abnormally:

    a.   low.
    b.   high.
    c.   neither a nor b.

31. (a,477)

31. The level of T_4 in Graves disease are usually abnormally:

    a.   high
    b.   low
    c.   neither a nor b

32. (d,477)

32. Upon palpation of Julia's neck, you would usually expect to feel:

    a.   normal-sized thyroid.
    b.   small discrete thyroid nodule.
    c.   multiple discrete thyroid nodules.
    d.   diffuse thyroid enlargement.

33. (b,479)

33. A low level of TSH usually leads to _____ hypothyroidism.

    a.   primary
    b.   secondary
    c.   autoimmune
    d.   none of the above

34. (a,479)

34. If a person has hypothyroidism because of iodine insufficiency, this is _____ hypothyroidism.

    a.   primary
    b.   secondary
    c.   autoimmune
    d.   none of the above

35. (b,479)

35. The basal metabolic rate is unusually _____ with hypothyroidism.

    a.   high
    b.   low
    c.   steady

36. (e,482)

36. Diagnosing thyroid carcinoma may involve:

a. measurement of serum thyroid levels.
b. radioisotope scanning.
c. ultrasonography.
d. small-needle aspiration biopsy.
e. all of the above.

37. (d,482)

37. _____ hyperparathyroidism is characterized by elevated secretion of PTH.

a. Secondary
b. Primary
c. Tertiary
d. a and b

38. (c,483)

38. Hypoparathyroidism is most commonly caused by:

a. pituitary hyposecretion.
b. parathyroid adenoma.
c. parathyroid gland damage.
d. hypothalamic inactivity.

39. (b,483)

39. Julia has her thyroid removed. During the postoperative period, you note that her serum calcium is low. You will observe her for which of the following signs/symptoms?

a. muscle weakness and constipation
b. laryngeal spasms and hyperreflexia
c. abdominal pain
d. anorexia, nausea, and vomiting

40. (c,483)

40. The most probable cause of Julia's low serum calcium is:

a. hyperparathyroidism secondary to Graves disease.
b. myxedema secondary to surgery.
c. hypoparathyroidism due to surgical injury.
d. hypothyroidism due to lack of thyroid replacement.

41. (e,485-486)

41. Bobby, a 12-year-old male, is admitted with acute type 1 diabetes mellitus (DM). In order for this diagnosis to have been made, Bobby had which of the following pathophysiologic characteristics:

a. peak occurrrence between 11 and 13 years
b. strong association with HLA-DR4
c. a combination of environmental and genetic factors as the cause
d. hyperglycemia and hyperketonemia
e. all of the above

42. (c,484)

42. Bobby's pathophysiologic state is most probably the result of:

a. familial, single gene abnormality.
b. obesity.
c. a multifactorial trait (gene-environmental).
d. hyperglycemia from eating too many sweets.

43. (b,487)

43. The initial major signs and symptoms you would expect Bobby to exhibit include:

    a. recurrent infections, visual changes, fatigue, paresthesias, serum glucose fluctuations.
    b. polydipsia, polyuria, polyphagia, weight loss, fatigue, serum glucose fluctuations.
    c. vomiting; abdominal pain; sweet, fruity breath; dehydration; Kussmaul breathing; serum glucose above normal.
    d. weakness, vomiting, hypotension, mental confusion, apathy, serum glucose below normal.

44. (b,487)

44. Bobby, now age 14, is admitted with the following lab values: arterial pH 7.20; serum glucose 500 mg/dl; urine glucose and ketones 4+/strong; serum K^+ 2; serum Na^+ 130. His parents state that he has been sick with the "flu" for a week. What relationship do these values have with his insulin deficiency?

    a. Increased glucose utilization causes the shift of fluid from the intravascular to the intracellular space.
    b. Decreased insulin causes fatty acid use, ketone formation, metabolic acidosis, and solute diuresis.
    c. Increased glucose and fatty acids stimulate renal diuresis, electrolyte loss, and metabolic alkalosis.
    d. Increased insulin use results in protein catabolism, tissue wasting, respiratory acidosis, and electrolyte loss.

45. (c,489)

45. Bobby is sent home on insulin. During his gym class, he experiences hunger, lightheadedness, tachycardia, pallor, headache, and confusion for the first time. The most probable cause of these symptoms is:

    a. hyperglycemia due to incorrect insulin administration.
    b. dawn phenomenon due to eating a snack before bedtime.
    c. hypoglycemia due to increased exercise.
    d. Somogyi effect due to insulin sensitivity.

46. (a,487-488)

46. Susan, a 55-year-old obese patient, is admitted to the medical unit complaining of a blister on her foot that has not healed. She says it looks "dark and ugly." She indicates she didn't even realize the blister was there until she removed her shoe and found it was bloody. She states she has been feeling poorly with some chest heaviness. She explains that it is difficult for her to read because she has had frequent blurred vision. You would expect which of the following lab values?

    a. serum glucose elevated; serum cholesterol elevated
    b. serum glucose elevated; serum cholesterol normal
    c. serum glucose normal; serum cholesterol elevated
    d. serum glucose decreased; serum cholesterol decreased

47. (c,491-493)

47. Susan is most likely experiencing which of the following complications of diabetes mellitus?

    1. diabetic neuropathy   5. microvascular disease
    2. peripheral vascular disease   6. retinopathy
    3. infection   7. nephropathy
    4. coronary artery disease

    a. 1, 3, 5, and 7
    b. 2, 4, 5, and 6
    c. 1, 2, 3, and 4
    d. 4, 5, 6, and 7

48. (c,494,497) 48. When differentiating Cushing syndrome and Addison disease, both usually have elevated levels of ACTH. However, Cushing syndrome has _____ levels of cortisol, and Addison disease has _____ levels of cortisol.

    a. elevated; normal
    b. decreased; elevated
    c. elevated; decreased
    d. decreased; normal

49. (d,494,498) 49. Hyperpigmentation as a result of increased ACTH may be seen in:

    a. Addison disease.
    b. Cushing disease.
    c. pheochromocytoma.
    d. a and b.
    e. all of the above.

Matching

50. (b,485) 50. ___ accounts for majority of cases   a. type 1 diabetes

51. (a,485) 51. ___ onset before age 30   b. type 2 diabetes

52. (b,485) 52. ___ obesity is a frequent characteristic

53. (b,485) 53. ___ incidence rising in U.S.

54. (a,485) 54. ___ 10% of all diabetes

55. (b,485) 55. ___ 90% of all diabetes

Short Answer

56. What are the three types of diabetes insipidus?

57. List one cause of primary and one cause of secondary hypothyroidism.

58. Most individuals with thyroid carcinoma have _____ T_3 and T_4 levels.

59. Kussmaul respirations occur in the following endocrine disorder:

60. Acne, moon face, purple striae, and trunkal obesity are seen in the following endocrine disorder:

Short Answers

56. Neurogenic, nephrogenic, psychogenic (473)
57. Primary: congenital defects, loss of thyroid tissue after hyperthyroidism treatment, defective hormone synthesis
    Secondary: insufficient stimulation of a normal gland, peripheral resistane to thyroid hormone (479)
58. Normal (482)
59. Diabetic ketoacidosis (489)
60. Cushing disease (494)

CHAPTER

19

Structure and Function of the Hematologic System

Name _____

True/False

1. (F,506)   1. T   F   Blood consists of a variety of formed elements, 60% water and 40% solutes.

2. (T,508)   2. T   F   Leukocytes are classified according to both structure and function.

3. (T,517)   3. T   F   If the body stores of iron are high and erythropoiesis is not increased, iron passes the plasma membrane of gut epithelial cells and is stored in the cells bound to ferritin. If the iron demand does not increase, the iron is excreted when the cells slough into the gut.

4. (T,513)   4. T   F   Erythropoietin is one of several colony-stimulating factors.

5. (T,513)   5. T   F   The kidneys secrete erythropoietin.

6. (T,521)   6. T   F   Thrombocytes develop from megakaryocytes by endomitosis.

7. (T,523)   7. T   F   Collagen attracts platelets out of the plasma.

8. (T,525)   8. T   F   Once activated, the clotting cascade is controlled by counteracting anticoagulants.

9. (F,514)   9. T   F   In adults, yellow bone marrow is normally active.

10. (T,526)   10. T   F   Breakdown of blood clots is carried out by the fibrinolytic system.

11. (F,527)   11. T   F   Aging causes major changes in blood composition.

Multiple Choice

12. (a,506)   12. The plasma proteins that are synthesized by lymphocytes in the lymph nodes are:

    a.   globulins.
    b.   albumins.
    c.   clotting factors.
    d.   complement proteins.

13. (e,506)

13. Which of the following are plasma proteins?

    a.   clotting factors
    b.   albumins
    c.   gamma globulins
    d.   immunoglobulins
    e.   all of the above

14. (c,508)

14. Two important characteristics allow erythrocytes to function as gas carriers. These are:

    a.   biconcavity and permanent shape.
    b.   permanent shape and reversible deformability.
    c.   reversible deformability and biconcavity.
    d.   biconcavity and the presence of hyperactive mitochondria.

15. (d,508)

15. All of the following are properties of erythrocytes *except*:

    a.   biconcavity.
    b.   reversible deformability.
    c.   presence of hemoglobin in cytoplasm.
    d.   presence of many mitochondria.

16. (c,509)

16. All of the following are granulocytes *except*:

    a.   neutrophils.
    b.   eosinophils.
    c.   monocytes.
    d.   basophils.
    e.   PMNs.

17. (d,509)

17. The _____ are granulocytes that contain granules of vasoactive amines.

    a.   neutrophils
    b.   eosinophils
    c.   monocytes
    d.   basophils

18. (b,510)

18. _____ are formed elements of the blood that are not cells, but disk-shaped cytoplasmic fragments essential for blood clotting.

    a.   Monocytes
    b.   Platelets
    c.   Macrophages
    d.   Erythrocytes

19. (d,508,510)

19. Which of the following formed elements of the blood do not undergo mitosis?

    a.   erythrocytes
    b.   platelets
    c.   macrophages
    d.   a and b
    e.   all of the above

20. (a,509)

20. _____ are blood cells that mature (differentiate) into macrophages.

    a. Monocytes
    b. Neutrophils
    c. Eosinophils
    d. Basophils

21. (a,511)

21. Which of the following is not a secondary lymph organ?

    a. thymus
    b. spleen
    c. tonsils
    d. Peyer's patches of the small intestine
    e. lymph nodes

22. (b,511)

22. All of the following are secondary lymphoid organs *except*:

    a. spleen
    b. bone marrow
    c. lymph nodes
    d. Peyer's patches
    e. tonsils

23. (a,513)

23. Which of the following is a site of fetal hemopoiesis?

    a. spleen
    b. gut
    c. Peyer's patches
    d. appendix

24. (d,511)

24. _____ proliferate in lymph nodes.

    a. Lymphocytes
    b. Monocytes
    c. Macrophages
    d. All of the above

25. (c,511-512)

25. Lymph enters the lymph nodes through several _____ lymphatic vessels, filters through the sinuses in the nodes, and leaves via _____ vessels.

    a. afferent, blood
    b. efferent, blood
    c. afferent, efferent lymphatic
    d. efferent, afferent lymphatic

26. (a,511)

26. During an infection, lymph nodes enlarge and become tender because:

    a. macrophages are rapidly dividing.
    b. the nodes are inflamed.
    c. the nodes are infected.
    d. the nodes are not functioning properly.

27. (a,511)

27. The process of hematopoiesis in the fetus differs from that in the adult. The differences include:

    a.   location.
    b.   initiation.
    c.   cessation.
    d.   induction and cessation.

28. (d,513)

28. Hematopoiesis occurs in the _____ of the fetus.

    a.   liver
    b.   bone marrow
    c.   spleen
    d.   a and c
    e.   all of the above

29. (d,513)

29. If there is a high demand on the hematopoietic system, medullary hematopoiesis can be accelerated by:

    a.   conversion of yellow bone marrow into red marrow.
    b.   faster differentiation of daughter cells.
    c.   faster proliferation of stem cells.
    d.   all of the above.

30. (e,513)

30. Colony-stimulating factors are regulatory molecules that stimulate the development of:

    a.   macrophages.
    b.   erythrocytes.
    c.   neutrophils.
    d.   a and c.
    e.   all of the above.

31. (b,515)

31. Which of the following shows a correct sequence in the development of erythrocytes?

    a.   normoblast, reticulocyte, basophilic erythroblast
    b.   polychromatophilic erythroblast, normoblast, reticulocyte
    c.   normoblast, committed proerythroblast, reticulocyte
    d.   normoblast, basophilic erythroblast, reticulocyte

32. (d,515)

32. All of the following are precursors to erythrocytes *except*:

    a.   hemopoietic stem cells.
    b.   normoblast.
    c.   megaloblast.
    d.   T cells.

33. (c,516)

33. Hemoglobin contains heme groups which allow it to carry oxygen. How many heme groups are present in hemoglobin?

    a.   two
    b.   three
    c.   four
    d.   five
    e.   eight

34. (b,517)

34. Erythropoietin:

    a. is secreted by the liver in response to tissue hypoxia.
    b. stimulates proliferation of stem cells.
    c. can cause a maximum production rate of 2.5 million erythrocytes per second.
    d. causes increased respiration in hypoxia.

35. (b,516)

35. Hemoglobin is a gene product and is therefore a:

    a. lipid.
    b. protein.
    c. carbohydrate.
    d. steroid.

36. (d,519)

36. Which of the following vitamins are needed for erythropoiesis?

    a. vitamin C and vitamin E
    b. vitamin B_{12} and vitamin B_2
    c. vitamin D and vitamin A
    d. a and b
    e. a, b, and c

37. (c,516)

37. _____ is an unstable type of hemoglobin that does not have the ability to bind oxygen.

    a. Deoxyhemoglobin
    b. Oxyhemoglobin
    c. Methemoglobin
    d. Glycosylated hemoglobin

38. (d,516)

38. About 70% of iron is bound to heme in:

    a. erythrocytes.
    b. hemosiderin.
    c. muscle cells.
    d. a and c.
    e. all of the above.

39. (b,518)

39. After erythrocytes have circulated for about 120 days, they are removed by macrophages of the MPS, which are chiefly in the:

    a. liver.
    b. spleen.
    c. appendix.
    d. bone marrow.

40. (a,521)

40. Hemostasis involves all of the following *except*:

    a. granulocytosis.
    b. blood clot formation.
    c. coagulation-cascade activation.
    d. platelet plug formation.
    e. vasoconstriction.

41. (c,525)

41. Which of the following shows a correct sequence in the coagulation cascade?

   a. X, tissue thromboplastin, XA
   b. prothrombin activator complex, X, XA
   c. damaged tissue, tissue thromboplastin, X
   d. fibrinogen, thrombin, tissue thromboplastin

42. (d,525)

42. Normal vascular epithelium prevents clotting because of:

   a. the texture of the endothelial lining.
   b. the negative charge of proteins in the endothelial cells.
   c. the presence of an anticlotting factor in the endothelial cells.
   d. a and b.
   e. a, b, and c.

43. (d,526)

43. All of the following are correct sequences in the fibrinolytic system *except*:

   a. plasminogen, plasmin.
   b. plasmin, fibrinogen.
   c. plasmin, fibrin.
   d. fibrin, plasminogen.

Ordering

44.

44. Number the following to show correct order

   (5,522)   ____   plug formation

   (6,522)   ____   clot retraction and dissolution

   (1,522)   ____   subendothelial exposure

   (4,522)   ____   aggregation

   (2,522)   ____   adhesion

   (3,522)   ____   activation

Short Answer

45. Plasma accounts for _____% of blood volume; formed elements account for

   _____%.

46. List the three plasma proteins.

47. What are the two unique properties of erythrocytes that make them ideal gas carriers.

48. List one primary and one secondary lymphoid organ.

49. What are the two stages of medullary hematopoiesis?

50. What is the normal lifespan of an erythrocyte?

Short Answers

45. 50 to 55; 45 to 50 (506)
46. Albumins, globulins, clotting factors (506)
47. Biconcavity, reversible deformity (508)
48. Primary: thymus, bone marrow
    Secondary: spleen, lymph nodes, tonsils, Peyer patches (511)
49. Proliferation and differentiation (513)
50. 80 to 120 days (508)

Alterations of Hematologic Function

Name _____

True/False

1. (F,536)

  1. T   F   When anemia is severe or sudden in onset, peripheral blood vessels dilate to direct blood flow to vital organs.

2. (T,538)

  2. T   F   Pernicious anemia is a form of megaloblastic anemia.

3. (T,538)

  3. T   F   Folate is essential for RNA synthesis.

4. (T,539)

  4. T   F   Iron deficient anemia is the most common type of anemia worldwide.

5. (T,539)

  5. T   F   The body may respond to a microbial infection by removing iron from the plasma (hypoferemia).

6. (T,547)

  6. T   F   The two major forms of leukemia, acute and chronic, are classified by predominant cell type.

7. (F,553,556)

  7. T   F   In both Hodgkin disease and non-Hodgkin lymphoma, T-cell function is severely decreased.

8. (F,553)

  8. T   F   Incidence rates of non-Hodgkin lymphoma do not differ with respect to age, gender, geographic location, and socioeconomic class.

9. (F,553)

  9. T   F   Philadelphia chromosome is present in multiple cells from the lymph nodes of an individual with Hodgkin disease.

10. (T,555)

  10. T   F   Frequently, the initial sign of Hodgkin disease is a painless mass, lump, or swelling most commonly on the neck.

11. (T,557)

  11. T   F   Splenomegaly can be primary, or it can be a secondary effect to other disorders in the body.

12. (T,561)

  12. T   F   One of the most common causes of disseminated intravascular coagulation, DIC, is malignancy.

13. (T,562)

  13. T   F   Disseminated intravascular coagulation is a paradoxical condition in which clotting and hemorrhage occur within the vascular system simultaneously.

Multiple Choice

14. (e,534)

14. Anemic conditions are caused by:

    a. impaired erythrocyte production.
    b. blood loss.
    c. increased erythrocyte destruction.
    d. a combination of impaired erythrocyte production, blood loss, and increased erythrocyte destruction.
    e. all of the above.

15. (b,539)

15. Erythrocytes that are _____ contain an abnormally low concentration of hemoglobin.

    a. hyperchromic
    b. hypochromic
    c. macrocytic
    d. none of the above

16. (c,534)

16. In some anemias the erythrocytes are present in various sizes; this is referred to as:

    a. normocytosis.
    b. isocytosis.
    c. anisocytosis.
    d. microcytosis.

17. (e,534-536)

17. A reduction in the number of circulating erythrocytes, such as seen after hemorrhage, affects the:

    a. viscosity of blood.
    b. speed of blood flow.
    c. turbulence of blood flow.
    d. hematocrit.
    e. all of the above.

18. (b,534)

18. Which of the following anemias is classified as a macrocytic normochromic anemia?

    a. iron deficiency anemia
    b. pernicious anemia
    c. sideroblastic anemia
    d. hemolytic anemia

19. (a,535)

19. Anemia causes arterioles, capillaries, and venules to _____, thus speeding the blood flow.

    a. dilate
    b. become compliant
    c. become noncompliant
    d. constrict

20. (c,535)

20. All of the following are normal adaptations to anemia *except*:

    a. increased rate and depth of breathing.
    b. increased cardiac output.
    c. decreased oxygen release from hemoglobin.
    d. blood vessels dilate.
    e. all of the above.

21. (a,536)	21. In megaloblastic anemia, erythrocytes contain _____ amounts of hemoglobin. a. normal b. sporadic c. low d. high
22. (a,536)	22. In macrocytic anemia, the cause is usually related in some way to: a. defective DNA synthesis. b. abnormal synthesis of hemoglobin. c. defective use of vitamin C. d. a and b. e. all of the above.
23. (c,528)	23. The underlying disorder of _____ anemia is defective secretion of intrinsic factor, which is essential for the absorption of vitamin B_{12}. a. microcytic b. hypochromic c. pernicious d. hemolytic
24. (c,538)	24. Untreated pernicious anemia is fatal, usually because of: a. brain hypoxia. b. liver hypoxia. c. heart failure. d. kidney failure.
25. (b,539)	25. Jimmy, an 18-month-old toddler weighing 28 pounds, is brought to the clinic because of weakness and sores at the corners of his mouth. His mother reports that the only food he will take is cow's milk. Considering this information, the nurse decides that Jimmy probably has: a. pernicious anemia. b. iron deficiency anemia. c. aplastic anemia. d. hemolytic anemia.
26. (b,539)	26. Which of the following clinical signs and symptoms would Jimmy most likely exhibit? a. hyperactivity b. pale palms and conjunctivae c. white tongue d. petechiae and purpura
27. (a,540)	27. Which of the following treatments would you expect to be prescribed for Jimmy? a. iron replacement and change of diet b. immediate transfusion of packed red blood cells c. a bone marrow transplant d. splenectomy and steroid therapy

28. (c,540)

28. Which of the following tests directly measures iron stores :

    a.   serum ferritin
    b.   transferrin saturation
    c.   bone marrow biopsy
    d.   total iron-binding capacity

29. (b,530)

29. Miss Green, a 58-year-old secretary, is seen in the clinic with complaints of chronic gastritis, fatigue, weight loss, and tingling in her fingers. Laboratory findings show a low hemoglobin and hematocrit, a high mean corpuscular volume, a normal plasma iron, and a high total iron-binding capacity and folate. These findings are consistent with which type of anemia?

    a.   folate deficiency anemia
    b.   pernicious anemia
    c.   iron deficiency anemia
    d.   aplastic anemia

30. (a,538)

30. The doctor orders the Schilling test to be given to Miss Green. This test involves:

    a.   administration of radioactive cobalamin and the measurement of its excretion in her urine.
    b.   the measurement of antigen-antibody immune complexes.
    c.   the measurement of serum ferritin and total iron-binding capacity.
    d.   the administration of folate and evaluation of folate content in a blood serum sample.

31. (b,538)

31. Which of the following treatments will probably be recommended for Miss Green?

    a.   B12 tablets
    b.   B12 injections
    c.   iron tablets
    d.   iron injections

32. (d,538)

32. How long will Miss Green need to continue this therapy?

    a.   a few weeks
    b.   a few months
    c.   until her iron level is normal
    d.   the rest of her life

33. (e,540)

33. Sideroblastic anemia is characterized by:

    a.   ineffective erythropoiesis caused by altered hemoglobin.
    b.   large numbers of sideroblast in the bone marrow.
    c.   increased levels of tissue iron.
    d.   varying proportions of hypochromic erythrocytes.
    e.   all of the above.

34. (a,540)

34. If a man has inherited the gene for sideroblastic anemia, he received it from his:

    a.   mother.
    b.   father.
    c.   mother and father.

35. (a,540)

35. A person with sideroblastic anemia would be likely to have:

    a.   iron overload.
    b.   pale skin.
    c.   normochromic erythrocytes.
    d.   aplastic bone marrow.

36. (c,540)	36. Clinical manifestations of iron overload may include all of the following *except*:

    a.   cardiac dysrythmias.
    b.   hepatomegaly.
    c.   atrophy of the spleen.
    d.   bronze-tinted skin.

37. (b,541)

37. Aplastic anemia is caused by:

    a.   iron deficiency.
    b.   folate deficiency.
    c.   vitamin B deficiency.
    d.   bone marrow hyperplasia.

38. (c,541)

38. In _____ anemia, splenectomy may be one of the treatments.

    a.   sideroblastic
    b.   megaloblastic
    c.   hemolytic
    d.   pernicious

39. (d,542)

39. All of the following pathogenic mechanisms cause anemia in chronic inflammation *except*:

    a.   decreased erythrocyte lifespan.
    b.   failure of mechanisms of compensatory erythropoiesis.
    c.   disturbances of the iron cycle.
    d.   increased basal metabolic rate.

40. (c,542)

40. Anemia of chronic inflammation is a mild to moderate anemia associated with chronic infections, chronic noninfectious inflammatory diseases, and malignancies. Chronic diseases commonly associated with this anemia include all of the following *except*:

    a.   rheumatoid arthritis.
    b.   Hodgkin disease.
    c.   polycythemia vera.
    d.   systemic lupus erythematosus.

41. (c,541)

41. Posthemorrhagic anemia can result in death when there is blood loss in excess of:

    a.   20–30%.
    b.   30–40%.
    c.   40–50%.
    d.   50–60%.

42. (b,534)

42. Normocytic-normochromic anemias include

    a.   sideroblastic anemia.
    b.   hemolytic anemia.
    c.   pernicious anemia.
    d.   iron deficiency anemia.

43. (c,542)

43. Mrs. Reaves, age 67, is admitted to the emergency room with a diagnosis of polycythemia vera. You expect her signs and symptoms to include:

    a.   hyperactivity.
    b.   decreased blood pressure.
    c.   chest pain.
    d.   a pale skin color.

44. (c,542) | 44. Mrs. Reaves' symptoms are mainly the result of:

   a. a decreased erythrocyte count.
   b. rapid blood flow to the major organs.
   c. increased blood viscosity.
   d. neurological involvement.

45. (a,543) | 45. Treatment for Mrs. Reaves might involve:

   a. therapeutic phlebotomy.
   b. restoration of blood volume by plasma expanders.
   c. the administration of packed red blood cells.
   d. iron replacement therapy.

46. (a,542) | 46. Excessively large numbers of erythrocytes in the blood is characteristic of:

   a. polycythemia vera.
   b. anemia.
   c. sideroblastic anemia.
   d. none of the above.

47. (a,543) | 47. The major cause of death in untreated polycythemia vera is:

   a. hemorrhage.
   b. renal failure.
   c. infection.
   d. leukemia.

48. (d,543) | 48. Polycythemia vera converts to_____in about 10% of individuals.

   a. chronic lymphocytic leukemia
   b. Burkitt lymphoma
   c. multiple myeloma
   d. acute myeloid leukemia

49. (b,543-544) | 49. Leukocytosis can be defined as:

   a. a normal leukocyte count.
   b. a higher leukocyte count.
   c. a lower leukocyte count.
   d. another term for leukopenia.

50. (b,543-544) | 50. _____ is a condition in which the leukocyte count is lower than normal.

   a. Leukocytosis
   b. Leukopenia
   c. Hypoleukocytosis
   d. None of the above

51. (e,544) | 51. Leukocytosis is a normal physiologic response to:

   a. invading microorganisms.
   b. emotional changes.
   c. temperature changes.
   d. pregnancy.
   e. all of the above.

52. (b,544) | 52. Clinically, neutropenia exists when the neutrophil count is less than _____ per milliliter.

    a. 5000
    b. 2000
    c. 1000
    d. 10,000

53. (e,544) | 53. Which of the following can cause eosinophilia?

    a. parasitic invasion
    b. dermatologic disorders
    c. allergic reactions
    d. a and c
    e. all of the above

54. (a,546) | 54. A patient is diagnosed with infectious mononucleosis. Which of the following is the predominant clinical manifestation?

    a. lymph node enlargement
    b. hepatitis
    c. rash on the trunk and extremities
    d. edema in the area of the eyes

55. (c,544) | 55. _____ is quite rare and, when present, is usually associated with hypersensitivity reactions of the immediate type.

    a. Eosinophilia
    b. Neutropenia
    c. Basophilia
    d. Basopenia

56. (b,546) | 56. Infectious mononucleosis is an acute infection of:

    a. monocytes.
    b. B lymphocytes.
    c. T lymphocytes.
    d. macrophages.

57. (e,546) | 57. The etiologic agent(s) of infectious mononucleosis is (are):

    a. cytomegalovirus.
    b. Epstein-Barr virus.
    c. Toxoplasma gondii.
    d. b and c.
    e. all of the above.

58. (c,547) | 58. Which of the following is a true statement?

    a. Only acute leukemias can be lymphocytic.
    b. Only chronic leukemias can be monocytic.
    c. Classification of leukemias has become increasingly complex.
    d. There are four principle types of chronic leukemias.

59. (e,549) 59. Which of the following represent clinical manifestations of acute leukemia?

   a. fever
   b. anorexia
   c. bleeding
   d. liver enlargement
   e. all of the above

60. (a,547) 60. _____ is a hereditary abnormality associated with an increased rate of leukemia.

   a. Down syndrome
   b. Hemophilia
   c. Hyperthyroidism
   d. Pheochromocytoma

61. (a,547) 61. _____ is an acquired disease that progresses to acute leukemia.

   a. Polycythemia vera
   b. Down syndrome
   c. Turner syndrome
   d. Klinefelter syndrome

62. (c,549) 62. _____ is the treatment of choice for leukemia.

   a. Bone marrow transplant
   b. Immunotherapy
   c. Chemotherapy
   d. None of the above

63. (b,551) 63. Multiple myeloma can be defined as a neoplasm of:

   a. T cells.
   b. B cells.
   c. immature plasma cells.
   d. mature red blood cells.

64. (e,553) 64. Reed-Sternberg cells are present in:

   a. acute leukemias.
   b. hemolytic anemia.
   c. thrombocytopenia.
   d. Hodgkin disease.

65. (b,553) 65. Enlarged lymph nodes (lymphadenopathy) can result from all of the following *except*:

   a. endocrine disorders.
   b. hypertensive disorders.
   c. lipid storage diseases.
   d. immunologic or inflammatory conditions.
   e. neoplastic disease.

66. (d,553) 66. Malignant lymphomas include:

   a. Hodgkin disease.
   b. non-Hodgkin lymphoma.
   c. multiple myeloma.
   d. a and b.

67. (c,553)   67. Hodgkin disease is characterized by an abnormal cell called:

   a. Merkel cell.
   b. Schwann cell.
   c. Reed-Sternberg cell.
   d. Kupffer cell.

68. (e,555)   68. The _____ lymph nodes are most commonly affected in Hodgkin disease, whereas the mesenteric epitrochlear, bronchial, and popliteal nodes are rarely involved.

   a. cervical
   b. axillary
   c. inguinal
   d. retroperitoneal
   e. all of the above

69. (d,557)   69. _____ is the virus associated with Burkitt lymphoma in African children.

   a. cytomegalovirus
   b. adenovirus
   c. human papilloma virus
   d. Epstein-Barr virus

70. (b,554)   70. The country with the lowest rate of Hodgkin disease is:

   a. the United States.
   b. Japan.
   c. Denmark.
   d. Great Britain.

71. (a,558)   71. Diffuse internal hemorrhage visible through the skin is known as:

   a. purpura.
   b. petechiae.
   c. ecchymosis.
   d. hemarthrosis.

72. (b,557)   72. Current criteria for hypersplenism include:

   a. Burkitt lymphoma.
   b. cellular bone marrow.
   c. infection.
   d. polycythemia vera.

73. (a,558)   73. Thrombocytopenia is a decreased_____count.

   a. platelet
   b. macrophage
   c. stem cell
   d. T-cell
   e. B-cell

74. (c,558) | 74. Thrombocytopenia may be:

    a. transient or consistent.
    b. normal or abnormal.
    c. primary or secondary.
    d. a and c.
    e. all of the above.

75. (b,558) | 75. Thrombocytopenia is described as a platelet count below _____ platelets per cubic millimeter.

    a. 1,000,000
    b. 100,000
    c. 10,000
    d. 1,000

76. (c,559) | 76. Primary thrombocythemia is a myeloproliferative disease in which _____ are overproduced.

    a. megakaryocytes
    b. reticulocytes
    c. platelets
    d. none of the above

77. (c,560) | 77. Vitamin _____ is required for normal clotting factor synthesis by the _____.

    a. K, kidneys
    b. D, kidneys
    c. K, liver
    d. D, liver

78. (b,560) | 78. The first clotting factor to decrease in liver disease is:

    a. factor II.
    b. factor VIII.
    c. factor X.
    d. factor IX.

79. (a,565) | 79. Which of the following is not a potential cause of thrombus formation?

    a. abnormal blood gases
    b. abnormal vessel wall
    c. abnormal blood flow
    d. altered blood constituents

Matching

80. (b,534) | 80. ____ thalassemia   a. macrocytic-normochromic

81. (c,534) | 81. ____ sickle cell anemia   b. microcytic-hypochromic

82. (a,534) | 82. ____ pernicious anemia   c. normocytic-normochromic

83. (c,534) | 83. ____ aplastic anemia

84. (c,534) | 84. ____ hemolytic anemia

85. (a,534) | 85. ____ folate deficiency anemia

86. (b,534) | 86. ____ iron deficiency anemia

Short Answer

87. List the components of Virchow triad.

88. What is the diagnostic marker for chronic myelocytic leukemia?

89. List the three goals of treatment for disseminated intravascular coagulopathy.

90. List two of the four types of conditions that cause lymphadenopathy.

Short Answers

87. (1) Injury to blood vessel endothelium; (2) abnormalities of blood flow; (3) hypercoagulability of the blood (565)
88. The Philadelphia chromosome (549)
89. (1) Removal of the underlying pathological condition; (2) restoration of an appropriate balance between coagulation and fibrinolysis; (3) maintaining organ viability (564)
90. (1) Neoplastic disease; (2) immunologic or inflammatory conditions; (3) endocrine disorders; (4) lipid storage diseases (553)

Alterations of Hematologic Function in Children

Name _____

True/False

1. (T,572)   1. T   F   Anemia is the most common blood disorder in children.

2. (T,572)   2. T   F   The most common cause of anemia in children is an iron deficiency.

3. (T,572)   3. T   F   The most dramatic form of aquired congenital hemolytic anemia is hemolytic disease of the newborn, also termed erythroblastosis fetalis.

4. (F,572)   4. T   F   Hemolytic disease of the newborn can occur only if antigens on fetal erythrocytes do not differ from antigens on maternal erythrocytes.

5. (T,572)   5. T   F   Rh incompatibility occurs in fewer than 10% of pregnancies and rarely causes hemolytic disease of the newborn in the first incompatible fetus.

6. (F,572)   6. T   F   G-6-PD is a defect of hemoglobin synthesis.

7. (T,576)   7. T   F   Sickled erythrocytes (characteristic of sickle cell anemia) tend to plug the micro-circulation.

8. (T,584)   8. T   F   The blast cell is the hallmark of acute leukemia.

9. (F,584)   9. T   F   Generally, girls are more likely to be diagnosed with a malignant lymphoma.

Multiple Choice

10. (c,572)   10. Iron deficiency anemia:

   a.   is most common between the ages of two and four.
   b.   is related to gender and race.
   c.   may be related to socioeconomic factors.
   d.   a and c.
   e.   all of the above.

11. (d,572)   11. Between age 4 and puberty, iron deficiency is:

   a.   frequently seen.
   b.   almost universal.
   c.   absent.
   d.   uncommon.

12. (e,583)   12. Childhood leukemia may be caused by:

    a.   genetic susceptibility.
    b.   environmental factors.
    c.   viral infections.
    d.   a and b.
    e.   all of the above.

13. (d,585)   13. Which condition increases the risk for malignant lymphoma?

    a.   sickle cell disease
    b.   sickle cell trait
    c.   renal failure
    d.   renal transplant

14. (c,585)   14. Hodgkin disease:

    a.   is frequently seen in children.
    b.   is more common in females than males.
    c.   may have an infectious mode of transmission.
    d.   has the same pathogenesis in children as in adults.

15. (b,572)   15. The most common cause of anemia from insufficient erythropoiesis in children is:

    a.   genetic factors.
    b.   iron deficiency.
    c.   hemoglobin abnormality.
    d.   erythrocyte structural abnormality.

16. (e,572)   16. Childhood hemolytic anemias can be:

    a.   inherited.
    b.   congenital.
    c.   acquired.
    d.   a and b.
    e.   all of the above.

17. (d,579)   17. Hydrops fetalis may result from which type of thalessemia?

    a.   beta minor
    b.   beta major
    c.   alpha minor
    d.   alpha major

18. (b,581)   18. Hemophilia B is also known as:

    a.   classic hemophilia.
    b.   Christmas disease.
    c.   thalassemia.
    d.   von Willebrand disease.

19. (a,572)   19. Which of the following is the most frequent blood disorder of infancy and childhood?

    a.   iron deficiency anemia
    b.   pernicious anemia
    c.   folate deficiency anemia
    d.   sideroblastic anemia

20. (c,572)

20. Intracellular defects of erythrocytes that result in premature removal of the erythrocytes from the circulation may include all of the following *except*:

   a. sickle cell disease.
   b. thalassemia.
   c. spherocytosis.
   d. G-6-PD deficiency.

21. (a,572)

21. When the hemoglobin content falls below _____ g/dl, tissue-compensatory mechanisms can no longer compensate adequately, and clinical manifestations of anemia become readily apparent.

   a. 5
   b. 8
   c. 12
   d. 14

22. (b,573)

22. Megaloblastic anemia in children may be caused by a deficiency of:

   a. vitamin K.
   b. vitamin B.
   c. vitamin C.
   d. vitamin E.

23. (b,572)

23. Hemolytic disease of the newborn can occur if:

   a. mother is Rh positive and fetus is Rh negative.
   b. mother is Rh negative and fetus is Rh positive.
   c. mother has type A blood and fetus has type O.
   d. mother has type AB blood and fetus has type B.

24. (b,572)

24. Maternal-fetal blood incompatibility may exist in which of the following conditions?

   a. mother Rh positive, fetus Rh negative
   b. mother Rh negative, fetus Rh positive
   c. father Rh negative, mother Rh positive
   d. father Rh negative, mother Rh negative

25. (b,572)

25. Erythroblastosis fetalis may be defined as:

   a. an allergic disease in which maternal and fetal blood are antigenically incompatible.
   b. an alloimmune disease in which maternal and fetal blood are antigenically incompatible.
   c. an autoimmune disease in which maternal and fetal blood are antigenically incompatible.
   d. b and c.
   e. all of the above.

26. (e,573)

26. Given that the mother and fetus have antigenically incompatible erythrocytes, hemolytic disease of the newborn will result if:

   a. maternal blood contains preformed antibodies directed against fetal erythrocyte antigen.
   b. sufficient amounts of antibodies cross the placenta.
   c. enough antibody binds to a sufficient number of fetal erythrocytes to cause extensive hemolysis.
   d. a and b.
   e. all of the above.

27. (b,574)

27. Fetuses that do not survive anemia in utero are usually stillborn, with gross edema of the entire body, a condition called:

    a.   hyperbilirubinemia.
    b.   hydrops fetalis.
    c.   erythroblastosis fetalis.
    d.   none of the above.

28. (a,575)

28. If excessive levels of bilirubin remain in the newborn, bilirubin will be deposited in the brain, a condition termed:

    a.   kernicterus.
    b.   icterus neonatorum.
    c.   jaundice.
    d.   hyperbilirubinemia.

29. (c,582)

29. The most serious complication of idiopathic thrombocytopenic purpura is:

    a.   respiratory infection.
    b.   asymmetric bruising.
    c.   intracranial bleeding.
    d.   immunosuppression.

30. (a,583)

30. Acute lymphoblastic leukemia:

    a.   is the most common childhood cancer.
    b.   affects nonwhite children twice as often as white children.
    c.   is seen more frequently seen in girls.
    d.   is rarely seen prior to age six.

31. (c,577)

31. Children with sickle cell disease:

    a.   have symptoms from the time of birth.
    b.   have a normal life expectancy.
    c.   most frequently die from infection.
    d.   can be successfully treated with medication.

32. (e,583)

32. Factors which increase the risk for childhood leukemia include:

    a.   radiation of the mother before conception.
    b.   prenatal radiation of the child.
    c.   maternal history of miscarriage.
    d.   early viral illness in the child.
    e.   all of the above.

33. (a,575)

33. Sickle cell disease is characterized by the presence of Hb S. Which of the following amino acids is present in Hb S and not present in normal Hb?

    a.   valine
    b.   glutamic acid
    c.   proline
    d.   histidine

34. (d,575) | 34. Which of the following is a true statement?

a. Sickle cell disease is an autosomal dominant disorder.
b. Sickle cell disease is an X-linked recessive disorder.
c. Sickle cell disease is an X-linked dominant disorder.
d. Sickle cell disease is an autosomal recessive disorder.

35. (b,575) | 35. Sickle cell disease is inherited in an _____ fashion.

a. autosomal dominant
b. autosomal recessive
c. X-linked dominant
d. X-linked recessive
e. none of the above; sickle cell disease is not clearly a genetic disease.

36. (c,575) | 36. If a person inherited sickle cell anemia, she most likely inherited it from:

a. her mother.
b. her father.
c. both her mother and father.
d. none of the above; sickle cell disease is not clearly an inherited disease.

37. (d,576) | 37. Erythrocytes of a person with sickle cell anemia may become sickled if:

a. oxygen tension is low.
b. pH is decreased.
c. plasma osmolality is increased.
d. all of the above.

38. (d,580) | 38. Classic hemophilia (hemophilia A) involves a deficiency in:

a. factor IX.
b. factor XII.
c. factor XIII.
d. factor VIII.
e. a and c.

39. (d,577) | 39. The type of sickle cell crisis seen only in young children is:

a. hyperhemolytic.
b. vasoocclusive.
c. aplastic.
d. sequestration.

40. (a,577) | 40. The alpha and beta thalassemias are inherited in an _____ fashion.

a. autosomal recessive
b. autosomal dominant
c. X-linked recessive
d. X-linked dominant

41. (c,577) | 41. If a male inherited an alpha-thalassemia, he most likely inherited it from his:

a. father.
b. mother.
c. mother and father.

42. (b,579)

42. Which form(s) of alpha-thalassemia is (are) fatal?

    a.   alpha-thalassemia minor
    b.   alpha-thalassemia major
    c.   hemoglobin H disese
    d.   a and b
    e.   a, b, and c

43. (c,582)

43. Idiopathic thrombocytopenic purpura (ITP) involves antibodies against:

    a.   neutrophils.
    b.   eosinophils.
    c.   platelets.
    d.   basophils.

Matching

44. (c,581)

44. ___ autosomal recessive   a. hemophilia A

45. (a,581)

45. ___ classic hemophilia   b. hemophilia B

46. (d,581)

46. ___ autosomal dominant   c. hemophilia C

47. (b,581)

47. ___ Christmas disease   d. von Willebrand disease

Short Answer

48. What are the four types of crisis that can occur in sickle cell anemia?

49. At one year following ITP, what percentage of affected children have normal platelet counts?

50. What is the most common symptom of Hodgkin disease in children?

Short Answers

48. 1. Vasocclusive (thrombotic) crisis
    2. Sequestration crisis
    3. Aplastic crisis
    4. Hyperhemolytic crisis (576-577)
49. 80% to 90% (582)
50. Painless adenopathy of the lower cervical chain, with or without fever (586)

Structure and Function of the Cardiovascular and Lymphatic Systems

Name _____

True/False

1. (T,590)

1. T   F   The heart pumps blood through two separate circulatory systems.

2. (F,590)

2. T   F   The adult heart weighs about two pounds.

3. (F,598)

3. T   F   To produce an action potential, the sinoatrial node must be stimulated by the autonomic nervous system.

4. (T,609)

4. T   F   The elastic arteries are more compliant than the muscular arteries.

5. (F,614)

5. T   F   Veins are less compliant than arteries.

6. (F,619)

6. T   F   Angiotensin II is the substrate for renin.

Multiple Choice

7. (c,590)

7. Judith Anderson is admitted to the cardiac unit with a diagnosis of pericarditis. She asks the nurse to explain where the infection is. In providing an accurate description, the nurse states that the pericardium is:

a.   the outer muscular layer of the heart.
b.   the innermost thin lining of the heart.
c.   a double-walled membranous sac that encloses the heart.
d.   the thick muscular layer of the heart which provides pumping action.

8. (d,590)

8. Functions of the pericardium include all of the following *except*:

a.   providing a physical barrier against extracardial infections and inflammations.
b.   affecting heart rate.
c.   affecting blood pressure.
d.   assisting in cardiac contraction.

9. (c,590)

9. The chamber of the heart that endures the highest pressures is the:

a.   right atrium.
b.   left atrium.
c.   left ventricle.
d.   right ventricle.

10. (b,590)   10. The chamber that is shaped like a crescent and acts like a bellows is the:

    a.   right atrium.
    b.   right ventricle.
    c.   left atrium.
    d.   left ventricle.

11. (b,594)   11. During diastole _____ valve(s) are/is open.

    a.   the semilunar
    b.   the atrioventricular
    c.   neither
    d.   both

12. (b,593)   12. The papillary muscles function to:

    a.   close the semilunar valves.
    b.   prevent backward expulsion of the atrioventricular valves.
    c.   close the atrioventricular valves.
    d.   prevent backward expulsion of the semilunar valves.

13. (c,598)   13. The heart is innervated by:

    a.   the sympathetic nervous system.
    b.   the parasympathetic nervous system.
    c.   both systems.
    d.   neither system.

14. (b,591)   14. Oxygenated blood flows through the:

    a.   superior vena cava.
    b.   pulmonary veins.
    c.   pulmonary artery.
    d.   coronary veins.

15. (a,593)   15. _____ are the anchors of the atrioventricular valves.

    a.   Chordae tendinae cordis
    b.   Great vessels
    c.   Coronary ostia
    d.   Trabeculae carneae cordis

16. (d,595)   16. The coronary ostia (the beginning of the coronary circulation) may be found in the:

    a.   left ventricle.
    b.   inferior vena cava.
    c.   coronary sinus.
    d.   aorta.
    e.   inferior vena cava.

17. (c,595)   17. The _____ is also called the anterior interventricular artery.

    a.   right coronary artery
    b.   left coronary artery
    c.   left anterior descending artery
    d.   circumflex artery

18. (a,597)

18. The coronary sinus empties into the:

    a. right atrium.
    b. left atrium.
    c. right ventricle.
    d. left ventricle.

19. (c,595)

19. The ratio of coronary capillaries to cardiac muscle cells is:

    a. many muscle cells per capillary.
    b. many capillaries per muscle cell.
    c. about one capillary per one muscle cell.
    d. about one capillary per 10 muscle cells.

20. (d,601)

20. The cardiac electrical impulse normally begins spontaneously in the SA node because:

    a. of its superior location in the right atrium.
    b. it is the only area of the heart capable of spontaneous depolarization.
    c. it has rich sympathetic innervation via the vagus nerve.
    d. it depolarizes more rapidly than other automatic cells of the heart.

21. (c,599)

21. The _____ supplies action potentials to the left posterior papillary muscles.

    a. Bachmann's bundle
    b. left anterior bundle branch
    c. left posterior bundle branch
    d. right bundle branch

22. (d,600)

22. _____ is an ion directly involved in the propagation of a cardiac action potential.

    a. Potassium
    b. Sodium
    c. Magnesium
    d. a and b
    e. All of the above

23. (b,599)

23. Depolarization of a cardiac muscle cell occurs as the result of a:

    a. decrease in the permeability of the cell membrane to ions.
    b. rapid movement of ions across the cell membrane.
    c. blockade by calcium ions.
    d. stimulus instigated during the refractory period.

24. (c,600)

24. In the normal electrocardiogram, the P-R interval represents:

    a. atrial depolarization.
    b. ventricular depolarization.
    c. onset of atrial to onset of ventricular activity.
    d. "electrical systole" of the ventricles.

25. (a,600)

25. The _____ follows depolarization of the myocardium and represents a period during which no new cardiac potential can be propagated.

    a. refractory period
    b. hyperpolarization period
    c. AV period
    d. SA period

26. (b,601)

26. The _____ represents the sum of all ventricular muscle cell depolarization.

   a. PR interval
   b. QRS
   c. QT interval
   d. P wave

27. (d,601)

27. Cells of the myocardium that normally have the property of spontaneous depolarization are found in the:

   a. aortic arch
   b. AV node.
   c. SA node.
   d. b and c.
   e. all of the above.

28. (b,601)

28. _____ nerves can shorten the conduction time of action potential's AV node.

   a. Parasympathetic
   b. Sympathetic
   c. Vagal
   d. Demylineated

29. (d,601)

29. The effect of acetylcholine on the heart is to:

   a. decrease the refractory period.
   b. increase calcium influx.
   c. increase the strength of myocardial contraction.
   d. decrease the heart rate.

30. (b,602)

30. _____ are thickened areas of the sarcolemma of myocardial cells that enable electrical impulses to travel in a continuous cell-to-cell fashion.

   a. Sarcolemma sclerotic plaques
   b. Intercalated discs
   c. Crossbridges
   d. A-bands

31. (c,604)

31. _____ is the process by which an action potential in the plasma membrane of a myocardial cell triggers the events that directly cause contraction of the myocardial cells.

   a. Electrocontraction
   b. Intercalated communication
   c. Excitation-contraction coupling
   d. Myosin communication

32. (a,605)

32. Within a physiologic range, an increase in left ventricular end diastolic volume (preload) leads to:

   a. an increase in cardiac output and an increased force of contraction.
   b. a decrease in cardiac output and a decreased force of contraction.
   c. an increase in cardiac output and a decreased force of contraction.
   d. a decrease in cardiac output and an increased force of contraction.

33. (a,606)   33. _____ is the pressure generated at the end of diastole.

    a. Preload
    b. Afterload
    c. Systemic vascular resistance
    d. Total peripheral resistance

34. (b,605)   34. As stated by the Frank-Starling law, there is a direct relationship between the _____ of the blood in the heart at the end of diastole and the _____ of contraction during the next systole.

    a. pressure, strength
    b. volume, force
    c. viscosity, force
    d. viscosity, strength

35. (e,606)   35. Pressure in the left ventricle must exceed pressure in the _____ before the left ventricle can eject blood.

    a. superior vena cava
    b. coronary sinus
    c. inferior vena cava
    d. pulmonary veins
    e. aorta

36. (b,606-607)   36. The resting heart in a healthy person is primarily under the control of the _____ nervous system.

    a. sympathetic
    b. parasympathetic
    c. somatic
    d. spinal

37. (a,607)   37. The Bainbridge reflex:

    a. increases heart rate following intravenous infusions.
    b. decreases blood pressure in response to pressoreceptors.
    c. increases rate and depth of respiration.
    d. decreases myocardial contractility.

38. (e,605)   38. Factors that affect cardiac performance include:

    a. preload.
    b. afterload.
    c. heart rate.
    d. myocardial contractility.
    e. all of the above.

39. (b,616)   39. Reflex control of total cardiac output and total peripheral resistance is controlled by:

    a. parasympathetic control of the heart, arterioles and veins.
    b. sympathetic control of the heart, arterioles and veins.
    c. autonomic control of the heart only.
    d. somatic control of the heart, arterioles and veins.

40. (c,621)

40. Myogenic regulation of blood vessel diameter and thus blood flow through a vessel is an example of _____ blood vessels.

   a. autonomic
   b. somatic
   c. autoregulation of
   d. metabolic regulation of

41. (d,616)

41. Baroreceptors are located in:

   a. the aorta.
   b. the vena cava.
   c. the carotid sinus.
   d. a and c.
   e. all of the above.

42. (c,622)

42. The coronary vessels are directly innervated by the _____ branch of the autonomic nervous system.

   a. sympathetic
   b. parasympathetic
   c. a and b
   d. none of the above

43. (a,623)

43. The major protein in lymph is:

   a. albumin.
   b. fibrinogen.
   c. complement.
   d. plasminogen.

44. (d,623)

44. The thoracic duct drains into the:

   a. right subclavian artery.
   b. right atrium.
   c. right subclavian vein.
   d. left subclavian vein.

45. (c,597)

45. Venous blood from the coronary circulation drains into the:

   a. superior vena cava.
   b. inferior vena cava.
   c. right atrium.
   d. left atrium.

46. (a,601)

46. Differences between cardiac and skeletal muscle include:

   a. cardiac muscle cells are arranged in branching networks.
   b. skeletal muscle cells have only one nucleus.
   c. cardiac muscle cells appear striped.
   d. skeletal muscle contains sarcomeres.

47. (e,602,604)

47. Myocardial oxygen consumption is determined by:

   a. amount of wall stress during systole.
   b. duration of systolic wall tension.
   c. contractile state of the myocardium.
   d. a and c.
   e. all of the above.

Matching

48. (e,593)

48. ____ semilunar valve

49. (b,593)

49. ____ atrioventricular valve

50. (d,593)

50. ____ annuli fibrosa cordis

51. (c,588)

51. ____ chordae tendineae cordis

52. (a,595)

52. ____ coronary ostia

a. openings in the aorta through which blood flows to the coronary arteries

b. mitral valve

c. structures which attach the atrioventricular valves to the papillary muscles

d. fibrous rings to which heart valves are attached

e. pulmonic valve

Short Answer

53. What do the following represent: P wave, P-R interval, QRS complex, Q-T interval, S-T interval, T wave.

54. What are the actions of the three components of the troponin complex?

55. What three factors determine myocardial oxygen consumption?

Short Answers

53. P wave—atrial depolarization; P-R interval—onset of atrial to onset of ventricular activity; QRS complex—ventricular depolarization; Q-T interval—electrical systole of the ventricles; S-T interval—period of entire ventricular depolarization; T wave—ventricular repolarization (600-601)

54. Troponin-T aids in binding the troponin complex to actin and tropomyosin.
    Troponin-I inhibits the atpase of actomyosin.
    Troponin-C contains binding sites for calcium ions involved in contraction. (602)

55. (1) Amount of wall stress during systole (measured by systolic blood pressure); (2) duration of systolic wall tension (measured by heart rate); (3) contractile state of the myocardium (no measurement possible) (602-604)

Alterations of Cardiovascular Function

Name _____

True/False

1. (F,638)

2. (T,638)

3. (T,640)

4. (F,639)

5. (F,641)

6. (F,641)

7. (T,630)

8. (T,633)

9. (T,645)

10. (F,648)

11. (T,655)

12. (T,660)

13. (T,672)

1. T   F   Orthostatic hypotension is compensated for solely by an increase in the contractility of the heart.

2. T   F   An aneurysm is a localized dilatation or outpouching of a blood vessel wall or cardiac chamber.

3. T   F   Even though air is lighter than blood, it can form an embolism and cause the occlusion of a blood vessel.

4. T   F   The pathophysiology of thrombus formation in veins is different than that in arteries.

5. T   F   Raynaud disease is characterized by vasospasms of coronary arteries.

6. T   F   Chronic venous insufficiency can progress to varicose veins and valvular incompetence.

7. T   F   Atherosclerosis is the leading contributor to coronary artery and cerebrovascular disease.

8. T   F   Prevalence rates for hypertensive disease are higher in men under 50 and women over 50.

9. T   F   Angina pectoris is chest pain caused by myocardial ischemia.

10. T   F   Percutaneous transluminal coronary angioplasty is generally employed only if a person has more than one stenotic coronary artery.

11. T   F   Pericardial effusion, even if in large amounts, does not necessarily result in cardiac tamponade.

12. T   F   Rheumatic fever is an inflammatory disease that results from a delayed immune response to a streptococcal infection.

13. T   F   An increase in left ventricular end diastolic volume may lead to pulmonary edema.

Multiple Choice

14. (a,629-630)   14. The fatty streak, an atherosclerotic lesion, causes_____obstruction of the affected vessel.

    a. no
    b. total
    c. intermittent
    d. partial

15. (d,629)   15. Arteriosclerosis raises the systolic pressure by:

    a. increasing arterial distensibility and lumen diameter.
    b. increasing arterial distensibility and decreasing lumen diameter.
    c. decreasing arterial distensibility and increasing lumen diameter.
    d. decreasing arterial distensibility and lumen diameter.

16. (a,633)   16. Most cases of combined systolic and diastolic hypertension have no known cause and are therefore diagnosed as _____ hypertension.

    a. primary
    b. secondary
    c. congenital
    d. acquired

17. (e,633)   17. Factors associated with primary hypertension include all of the following *except*:

    a. family history of hypertension.
    b. black race.
    c. high dietary sodium intake.
    d. cigarette smoking.
    e. preeclampsia.

18. (b,633)   18. All of the following represent risk factors for primary hypertension *except*:

    a. family history of hypertension.
    b. high potassium intake.
    c. black race.
    d. increased alcohol consumption.
    e. male gender.

19. (d,633)   19. Elevations of systolic pressure alone are usually caused by:

    a. increases in cardiac output.
    b. rigidity of the aorta.
    c. high sodium intake.
    d. a and b.
    e. all of the above.

20. (a,633)   20. Localized dilation or outpouching of a vessel wall or cardiac chamber is called:

    a. aneurysm.
    b. thrombus.
    c. embolus.
    d. thromboembolus.

21. (c,638)

21. Cerebral aneurysms frequently occur in the:

    a.   vertebral arteries.
    b.   basilar artery.
    c.   circle of Willis.
    d.   carotid arteries.

22. (c,639)

22. A detached blood clot is called a:

    a.   thrombus.
    b.   embolus.
    c.   thromboembolus.
    d.   varicosity.

23. (a,640)

23. _____ is the obstruction of a blood vessel by an embolus.

    a.   Embolism
    b.   Plaque
    c.   Aneurysm
    d.   Varicosity

24. (e,640)

24. Which of the following is a source of emboli?

    a.   amniotic fluid
    b.   fat
    c.   bacteria
    d.   b and c
    e.   all of the above

25. (e,640)

25. Which of the following does not form an embolism?

    a.   amniotic fluid
    b.   bacteria
    c.   fat
    d.   air
    e.   ischemia

26. (d,641)

26. _____ is characterized by attacks of vasospasm in the small arteries and arterioles of the fingers and, less commonly, the toes.

    a.   Raynaud phenomenon
    b.   Raynaud disease
    c.   Buerger disease
    d.   a and b
    e.   all of the above

27. (e,641)

27. An individual is diagnosed with varicose veins. Which of the following is a possible cause?
    a.   action of gravity on blood
    b.   long periods of standing
    c.   trauma to the saphenous veins
    d.   a and b
    e.   all of the above

28. (b,642)

28. Superior vena cava syndrome is a progressive _____ of the superior vena cava that leads to venous distention of the upper extremities and head.

   a. inflammation
   b. obstruction
   c. distention
   d. sclerosis

29. (b,643)

29. Coronary artery disease can diminish the myocardial blood supply until deprivation impairs myocardial metabolism enough to cause _____, a local state in which the cells are temporarily deprived of blood supply.

   a. infarction
   b. ischemia
   c. necrosis
   d. angina

30. (b,633)

30. Of the following risk factors for coronary artery disease, which is most predictive of the disease?

   a. diabetes mellitus
   b. hypertension
   c. obesity
   d. high alcohol consumption

31. (c,631)

31. Dietary modification in arteriosclerosis includes decreasing daily fat intake to less than _____ of calories.

   a. 10%
   b. 20%
   c. 30%
   d. 40%

32. (a,643)

32. _____ is one of the most predictive risk factors for coronary heart disease.

   a. Dyslipidemia
   b. Diabetes insipidus
   c. Sex
   d. Diabetes mellitus

33. (a,645)

33. Cardiac cells can withstand ischemic conditions, and still return to a viable state, for:

   a. 20 minutes
   b. 25 minutes
   c. 30 minutes
   d. none of the above; cellular death is immediate with ischemic conditions

34. (c,645)

34. _____ angina occurs unpredictably and almost exclusively when the person is at rest.

   a. Unstable
   b. Crescendo
   c. Prinzmetal
   d. Acute coronary insufficiency

35. (b,647)

35. The aim of therapy for myocardial ischemia includes all of the following *except*:

a. increased ventricular volume.
b. increased systolic blood pressure.
c. decreased heart rate.
d. decreased myocardial oxygen demand.

36. (c,645)

36. Myocardial cells can withstand ischemic conditions for approximately _____ minutes before cellular death takes place.

a. 5
b. 10
c. 20
d. 40

37. (e,650)

37. Functional changes in the myocardium caused by myocardial infarction include:

a. altered left ventricular compliance.
b. decreased cardiac contractility with abnormal wall movement.
c. decreased stroke volume.
d. sinoatrial node dysfunction.
e. possibly all of the above.

38. (b,653)

38. Following myocardial infarction the first_____is the time of highest risk for sudden death.

a. hour
b. 24 hours
c. 48 hours
d. week

39. (b,651)

39. An individual is demonstrating elevated levels of creatine phosphate and lactic dehydrogenase. These elevated levels indicate:

a. Raynaud disease.
b. myocardial infarction.
c. orthostatic hypertension.
d. varicose veins.

40. (e,653)

40. Cardiac dysrhythmias may be caused by:

a. ischemia.
b. hypoxia.
c. autonomic nervous system imbalances.
d. abnormalities in potassium levels.
e. all of the above.

41. (a,655)

41. Pericardial effusion can cause cardiac compression known as:

a. tamponade.
b. exudate.
c. aneurysm.
d. pulsus paradoxus.

42. (e,655)   42. Currently, in the United States, constrictive pericarditis is often associated with:

    a.   radiation exposure.
    b.   rheumatoid arthritis.
    c.   uremia.
    d.   coronary bypass surgery.
    e.   all of the above.

43. (e,656)   43. Cardiomyopathies are categorized as:

    a.   dilated.
    b.   hypertrophic.
    c.   constrictive.
    d.   a and b.
    e.   all of the above.

44. (d,657)   44. Conditions that can cause dilated cardiomyopathy include:

    a.   alcoholism.
    b.   pregnancy.
    c.   muscle growth defect.
    d.   a and b.
    e.   all of the above.

45. (b,638)   45. Acute orthostatic hypotension is caused by:

    a.   endocrine disorders.
    b.   drug action.
    c.   idiopathic causes.
    d.   metabolic disorders.

46. (d,639)   46. A _____ aneurysm requires emergency repair.

    a.   saccular
    b.   circumferential
    c.   false
    d.   dissecting

47. (d,657)   47. In _____, the cardiac valve leaflets, or cusps, fail to shut completely, permitting blood flow even when the valve should be completely closed.

    a.   valvular regurgitation
    b.   valvular insufficiency
    c.   valvular incompetence
    d.   all of the above

48. (d,657)   48. _____ is (are) a common cause of aortic stenosis.

    a.   Inflammatory damage
    b.   Congenital malformation
    c.   Calcification
    d.   All of the above

49. (c,658)

49. Mitral stenosis results directly in the incomplete emptying of the:

   a.   right atrium.
   b.   right ventricle.
   c.   left atrium.
   d.   left ventricle.

50. (a,660)

50. _____ is the most common cardiac valve disease in the United States and tends to be most prevalent in young women.

   a.   Mitral valve prolapse
   b.   Tricuspid stenosis
   c.   Tricuspid valve prolapse
   d.   None of the above

51. (a,664)

51. Infective endocarditis is most often caused by:

   a.   bacteria.
   b.   viruses.
   c.   fungi.
   d.   parasites.

52. (d,664)

52. Risk factors for endocarditis include:

   a.   acquired valvular disease.
   b.   prosthetic heart valves.
   c.   turbulent cardiac blood flow.
   d.   all of the above.

53. (b,666)

53. Clinical manifestations of cardiac disease are seen in about _____% of those with HIV infections.

   a.   5-10
   b.   25-50
   c.   60-70
   d.   90-100

54. (c,675)

54. Right heart failure is commonly called:

   a.   congestive heart failure.
   b.   restrictive heart failure.
   c.   cor pulmonale.
   d.   biventricular heart failure.

55. (d,675)

55. High output failure:

   a.   causes metabolic alkalosis.
   b.   occurs with hypothyroidism.
   c.   occurs with hypovolemia.
   d.   in seen in septicemia.

56. (a,675)

56. A patient is diagnosed with pulmonary disease and elevated pulmonary vascular resistance. Which of the following heart failures may result from this condition?

   a.   right heart failure
   b.   left heart failure
   c.   low-output failure
   d.   high-output failure

57. (d,675)   57. High output cardiac failure is usually attributable to the _____ ventricle.

    a. left
    b. right
    c. Both ventricles are dysfunctional.
    d. Neither ventricle is dysfunctional.

58. (a,679)   58. Which of the following is not a type of shock?

    a. hormonal
    b. septic
    c. hypovolemic
    d. neurogenic

59. (e,680)   59. Shock may be classified by cause into each of the following categories *except*:

    a. cardiogenic.
    b. hypovolemic.
    c. neurogenic.
    d. anaphylactic.
    e. hepatic.

60. (e,680)   60. Hypovolemic shock may be initially compensated for by:

    a. epinephrine release from the adrenal glands.
    b. release of stored erythrocytes from the liver.
    c. release of stored erythrocytes from the spleen.
    d. an increase in systemic vascular resistance.
    e. all of the above.

61. (c,680)   61. Neurogenic shock can be caused by any factor that stimulates the _____ nervous system or inhibits the _____ nervous system.

    a. parasympathetic, somatic
    b. sympathetic, somatic
    c. parasympathetic, sympathetic
    d. sympathetic, parasympathetic

Matching

62. (d,659)   62. ___ rheumatic heart disease   a. seen with inherited connective tissue disorders

63. (a,660)   63. ___ mitral valve prolapse   b. edema of the upper extremities and face

64. (e,681)   64. ___ sepic shock   c. seen in heavy smokers and young men

65. (b,642)   65. ___ superior vena cava syndrome   d. aortic regurgitation

66. (c,640)   66. ___ Buergers disease   e. may progress to MODS

Short Answer

67. List three inflammatory mediators that contribute to septic shock.

68. What organ system is frequently the first to fail in MODS?

69. What route for nutrition is best for postoperative/posttrauma individuals?

70. Rheumatic heart disease follows infection of what organism?

Short Answers

67. The interleukins, tumor necrosis factor, platelet-activating factor, myocardial depressant factor (684)
68. Pulmonary system (687)
69. Enteral nutrition (688)
70. Group A ß-hemolytic streptococcus (661)

Alterations of Cardiovascular Function in Children

Name _____

True/False

1. (F,699)	1. T	F	Congenital heart disease is a major cause of death in the first year of life.
2. (F,703)	2. T	F	Closure of the ductus arteriosus normally occurs immediately after birth.
3. (F,705)	3. T	F	A systemic viral infection of rubella generally results in ventricular septal defect, a congenital heart defect.
4. (F,703)	4. T	F	The abnormal movement of blood from the pulmonary to the systemic circulation is called a left-to-right shunt.
5. (T,706)	5. T	F	Complete transposition of the great vessels is a congenital heart defect in which the left ventricle pumps blood to the pulmonary circulation.
6. (T,707)	6. T	F	In some cases of total anomalous pulmonary venous return, pulmonary veins drain into the vena cava.
7. (T,710-711)	7. T	F	The clinical manifestations of congestive heart failure in children include failure to thrive and periorbital edema.
8. (F,709)	8. T	F	In general the pathophysiologic mechanisms of congestive heart failure are very different in children than in adults.
9. (T,711)	9. T	F	Peripheral edema is common in adults with left heart failure, but rare in children with left heart failure.
10. (T,711)	10. T	F	Kawasaki disease is a cause of pediatric-acquired heart disease in the United States.
11. (F,712)	11. T	F	The pathophysiology of primary hypertension in children is clearly understood.
12. (F,712)	12. T	F	All hypertension in children is considered primary hypertension.

Multiple Choice

13. (d,700)

13. Coarctation of the aorta results in:

   a. warm legs.
   b. bounding pedal pulses.
   c. cool arms.
   d. weak or absent femoral pulses.

14. (c,703)

14. _____ is a patent opening between the aorta and pulmonary artery in a fetus.

   a. Foramen ovale
   b. Ductus venosus
   c. Ductus arteriosus
   d. Foramen magnum

15. (b,700)

15. Acyanotic heart defects:

   a. usually involve a right-to-left shunt.
   b. may have no shunt at all.
   c. result in bluish skin color.
   d. a and b.
   e. all of the above.

16. (b,699)

16. The incidence of congenital heart disease is:

   a. 4%–8%
   b. 0.4%–0.8%
   c. 14%–18%
   d. 1.4%–1.8%

17. (a,699-700)

17. All of the following represent genetic disorders that can lead to congenital heart defects except:

   a. Raynaud disease.
   b. trisomy 18.
   c. Down syndrome.
   d. Turner syndrome.

18. (a,700)

18. Congenital heart defects that cause hypoxia and therefore cyanosis usually involve _____ shunts.

   a. right-to-left
   b. left-to-right
   c. ductus venosus
   d. all of the above

19. (c,702)

19. Pulmonic stenosis is the narrowing of the:

   a. mitral valve.
   b. pulmonary artery.
   c. pulmonary semilunar valve.
   d. pulmonary vein.

20. (d,699)   20. Chromosomal abberations involved with CHD include:

             a. trisomy 13.
             b. trisomy 18.
             c. trisomy 21.
             d. all of the above.

21. (d,701)   21. Coarctation of the aorta:

             a. requires cardiac bypass for repair.
             b. can only be treated with surgery.
             c. should be electively repaired after age 2.
             d. has a recurrence risk.

22. (b,700)   22. All of the following are manifestations of aortic coarctation except:

             a. epistaxis.
             b. poor cranial blood supply.
             c. cyanosis of the lower extremities.
             d. decreased or absent femoral pulse.

23. (e,699)   23. Environmental factors that may be associated with congenital heart disease are:

             a. infections.
             b. radiation exposures.
             c. drugs.
             d. a and b.
             e. all of the above.

24. (b,705)   24. Atrioventricular canal defects are the most common cardiac defect in children with:

             a. rubella exposure in utero.
             b. Down syndrome.
             c. prematurity.
             d. cocaine exposure in utero.

25. (c,705)   25. Atrioventricular canal defect can be characterized by:

             a. the failure of the ductus arteriosus to close.
             b. fusion of the endocardial cushions.
             c. blood flow between all four heart chambers.
             d. right-to-left shunt.

26. (c,703)   26. Patent ductus arteriosus is caused by:

             a. viral infection.
             b. bacterial infection.
             c. an unknown mechanism.
             d. a and b.
             e. all of the above.

27. (a,709)   27. Hypoplastic left heart syndrome is:

             a. an indication for neonatal heart transplant.
             b. rarely fatal.
             c. easily repaired.
             d. asymptomatic.

28. (a,708)

28. The clinical manifestations of truncus arteriosus include:

    a.   left heart failure.
    b.   crackles in the lungs.
    c.   cyanosis.
    d.   a and b.
    e.   all of the above.

29. (a,706)

29. Which of the following is consistent with the cardiac defect of transposition of the great vessels?

    a.   The aorta arises from the right ventricle.
    b.   The pulmonary trunk arises from the right ventricle.
    c.   The right ventricle pumps blood to the lungs.
    d.   The left ventricle pumps blood to the body.

30. (c,708)

30. Complete transposition of the great vessels may be defined as:

    a.   total absence of capillaries.
    b.   total absence of arterioles.
    c.   the complete switching of the aorta and pulmonary arteries.
    d.   the abnormal entry of blood from the pulmonary circulation into the right atrium.

31. (b,706)

31. Which of the following describes total anomalous pulmonary venous return?

    a.   The foramen ovale closes after birth.
    b.   Pulmonary venous return is to the right atrium.
    c.   Pulmonary venous return is to the left atrium.
    d.   The foramen ovale does not close.

32. (e,705)

32. Tetrology of Fallot includes:

    a.   ventricular septal defect.
    b.   pulmonic stenosis.
    c.   overriding aorta.
    d.   right ventricular hypertrophy.
    e.   all of the above.

33. (a,712)

33. Secondary hypertension in children can be caused by:

    a.   kidney disease.
    b.   stress.
    c.   obesity.
    d.   high fat intake.

34. (a,711)

34. All of the following represent the most commonly acquired cardiovascular disorders of children except:

    a.   hypotension.
    b.   hypertension.
    c.   left heart failure.
    d.   rheumatic heart disease.

35. (d,711)	35. The cause of Kawasaki disease is clearly:

    a. genetic.
    b. viral.
    c. bacterial.
    d. not known.

Matching

36. (d,700)   36. ___ obstructive defect   a. patent ductus arteriosus

37. (a,703)   37. ___ defect with increased pulmonary blood flow   b. tetrology of Fallot

    c. cardiomyopathy

38. (d,705)   38. ___ defect with decreased pulmonary blood flow   d. coarctation of the aorta

39. (d,708)   39. ___ mixed defect   e. truncus arteriosus

40. (d,711)   40. ___ acquired disorder

Short Answer

41. List four signs and symptoms of Kawasaki disease.

42. List four environmental factors associated with congenital heart disease.

43. Why is valvular aortic stenosis serious?

44. What are the four defects in tetralogy of Fallot?

45. Describe the three types of truncus arteriosus.

Short Answers

41. Fever for five days or more, bilateral conjunctions without exudate, changes in oral mucous membranes, changes in extremities, polymorphous rash, cervical lymphadenopathy (711)
42. Infection, radiation, metabolic disorders, drugs, peripheral conditions (699)
43. (1) The obstruction tends to be progressive; (2) sudden episodes of myocardial ischemia or low cardiac output can result in sudden death; (3) surgical repair will not result in a normal value (702)
44. Ventricular septal defect, pulmonary stenosis, orverriding aorta, right ventricular hypertrophy (705)
45. Type I—a single pulmonary trunk arises near the base of the truncus and divides into the left and right pulmonary arteries.

    Type II—the left and right pulmonary arteries arise separately.

    Type III—the pulmonary arteries arise independently and from the lateral aspect of the truncus. (708)

CHAPTER

25

Structure and Function of the Pulmonary System

Name _____

True/False

1. (T,719)

1. T   F   The oropharynx is considered part of a conducting airway.

2. (T,721)

2. T   F   The trachea bifurcates into two bronchi at the carina.

3. (F,722)

3. T   F   While a person is resting, the entire pulmonary circulation is still perfused, although at a slower rate than during exercise.

4. (T,722)

4. T   F   Veins of the pulmonary circulation are similar to the veins of systemic circulation but contain no one-way valves.

Multiple Choice

5. (a,718)

5. The primary function of the pulmonary system is best described as:

a.   the exchange of gases between the environment and blood.
b.   the intake and expelling of air.
c.   the movement of blood into and out of the capillaries.
d.   the principle mechanism for cooling of the heart.

6. (a,718)

6. The movement of blood into and out of the capillary beds of the lungs to the body organs and tissues is called:

a.   perfusion.
b.   ventilation.
c.   diffusion.
d.   active transport.

7. (d,719)

7. The nasopharynx is lined with a ciliated mucosal membrane with a highly vascular blood supply. The function of the membrane is:

a.   to absorb air.
b.   to moisten air.
c.   to clean air.
d.   b and c.
e.   a, b, and c.

8. (a,719)

8. The slit-shaped space between the true vocal cords forms the:

    a. glottis.
    b. epiglottis.
    c. larynx.
    d. carina.

9. (e,719,721)

9. Laryngeal muscles:

    a. control voice pitch.
    b. prevent aspiration.
    c. assist in swallowing.
    d. a and c.
    e. a, b, and c.

10. (a,721)

10. Type I alveolar cells_____; type II alveolar cells_____.

    a. secrete surfactant; provide structure
    b. provide structure; secrete surfactant
    c. ingest foreign material; exchange gases
    d. exchange gases; ingest foreign material

11. (b,721)

11. All of the following may be found in the respiratory bronchioles *except*:

    a. smooth muscle.
    b. surfactant-producing glands.
    c. goblet cells.
    d. ciliated cells.

12. (c,721)

12. Surfactant produced by type II alveolar cells facilitates alveolar distention and ventilation by:

    a. decreasing thoracic compliance.
    b. attracting water to the alveolar surface.
    c. decreasing surface tension in alveoli.
    d. increasing diffusion in alveoli.

13. (d,721)

13. The gas exchange airways are made up of the:

    a. respiratory bronchioles.
    b. alveolar ducts.
    c. terminal bronchioles.
    d. a and b.
    e. a, b, and c.

14. (b,721)

14. _____ secrete surfactant, a lipoprotein that coats the inner surface of the alveoli.

    a. Type I alveolar cells
    b. Type II alveolar cells
    c. Alveolar macrophages
    d. All of the above

15. (e,723)

15. The alveolocapillary membrane is composed of:

    a. the alveolar basement membrane.
    b. the alveolar epithelium.
    c. the capillary basement membrane.
    d. the capillary endothelium.
    e. all of the above.

16. (c,723)   16. There are no lympahtic vessels associated with:

    a.   the entire lung.
    b.   bronchi.
    c.   alveoli.
    d.   terminal bronchioles.

17. (b,723)   17. The pleural membranes are examples of _____ membranes.

    a.   mucous
    b.   serous
    c.   synovial
    d.   peritoneal

18. (b,726)   18. Norms for lung volumes and capacities are based on:

    a.   age.
    b.   gender.
    c.   height.
    d.   all of the above.

19. (d,726)   19. Of the following measurements, which would you expect total lung capacity to be nearest?

    a.   3000 mls
    b.   4000 mls
    c.   5000 mls
    d.   6000 mls

20. (a,726)   20. The _____ is the maximum amount of gas that can be displaced (expired) from the lung.

    a.   vital capacity
    b.   total lung capacity
    c.   functional capacity
    d.   none of the above

21. (b,729)   21. During inspiration, muscular contraction of the diaphragm causes the size of the thorax to increase. This increased size causes a decrease in intrapleural pressure, causing:

    a.   air to move out of his lungs.
    b.   air to move into his lungs.
    c.   no air movement.

22. (b,733)   22. Approximately 1000 ml (1 liter) of oxygen is transported to cells each minute. Most of the oxygen is transported:

    a.   dissolved in his plasma.
    b.   loosely bound to his hemoglobin.
    c.   in the form of CO_2.
    d.   as a free-floating molecule.

23. (a,736)   23. In acidosis or a fever, you would expect the oxyhemoglobin dissociation curve to:

    a.   shift to the right, causing more O_2 to be released to the cells.
    b.   shift to the left, allowing less O_2 to be released to the cells.
    c.   show no change, allowing the O_2 concentration to remain stable.

24. (b,734)

24. If Mr. Jones' hemoglobin concentration (Hb) is 14 gms/100 mls and his arterial oxygen saturation (SaO_2) is 98%, what would be his arterial oxygen content? Remember 1.34 mls O_2 is the maximum amount of oxygen that can be transported per gram of hemoglobin. Hint: O_2 content = (1.34 x Hb) SaO_2.

    a.   13.72 mls O_2 per 100 mls blood
    b.   18.38 mls O_2 per 100 mls blood
    c.   18.76 mls O_2 per 100 mls blood
    d.   19.30 mls O_2 per 100 mls blood

25. (b,736)

25. The carbon dioxide in Mr. Jones' system is mainly carried in the blood:

    a.   attached to oxygen.
    b.   in the form of bicarbonate.
    c.   combined with albumin.
    d.   dissolved in RBCs.

26. (a,729)

26. The _____ is an accessory muscle of inspiration.

    a.   sternocleidomastoid
    b.   diaphragm
    c.   external intercostal
    d.   b and c
    e.   all of the above

27. (e,727)

27. The respiratory center is composed of several groups of neurons in the brain stem; included in these groups are all of the following except the:

    a.   dorsal respiratory group.
    b.   ventral respiratory group.
    c.   pneumotaxic center.
    d.   apneustic center.
    e.   chemoreceptors.

28. (a,727)

28. _____ are receptors in the lung that decrease ventilatory rate and volume.

    a.   Stretch receptors
    b.   Baroreceptors
    c.   Carbon dioxide receptors
    d.   Chemoreceptors

29. (a,727)

29. The lung is innervated by the parasympathetic nervous system via the _____ nerve.

    a.   vagus
    b.   phrenic
    c.   brachial
    d.   pectoral

30. (c,733)

30. At the base of the lungs:

    a.   alveolar gas pressure exceeds arterial perfusion pressure.
    b.   arterial perfusion pressure and alveolar gas pressure are less than at the apex.
    c.   arterial perfusion pressure exceeds alveolar gas pressure.
    d.   arterial perfusion and alveolar gas pressure are equal.

31. (a,733)

31. In the lung it takes _____ seconds for oxygen concentration to equilibrate across the alveolo capillary membrane:

   a. 0.25
   b. 2.5
   c. 0.75
   d. 7.5

32. (a,737)

32. Normal aging results in _____ lung compliance.

   a. increased
   b. decreased
   c. no change in
   d. absent

33. (e,730)

33. Airway resistance is determined by:

   a. length and radius of the airways.
   b. density of gas.
   c. velocity of gas.
   d. b and c.
   e. a, b, and c.

34. (b,727-728)

34. If Mr. Smith hypoventilates and retains too much carbon dioxide, which of the following receptors would be stimulated in an attempt by his body to maintain a normal homeostatic state?

   a. irritant receptors
   b. central chemoreceptors
   c. peripheral chemoreceptors
   d. stretch receptors

35. (a,727-728)

35. After these receptors were stimulated, you would expect Mr. Smith's respirations to:

   a. increase in rate.
   b. decrease in rate.
   c. remain the same.

Matching

36. (d,721)

36. ____ type I alveolar cells   a. secrete surfactant

37. (a,721)

37. ____ type II alveolar cells   b. monitor pH changes

38. (c,727)

38. ____ irritant receptors   c. sensitive to noxious stimuli

39. (e,727)

39. ____ stretch receptors   d. provide structure

40. (f,727)

40. ____ J-receptors   e. sensitive to increases in lung size and volume

41. (b,727)

41. ____ central chemoreceptors   f. sensitive to pulmonary capillary pressure

Short Answer

42. List the three steps in gas exchange.

43. List the three lung zones and give their locations.

44. What is the Bohr effect?

45. List the structures of the acinus.

Short Answers

42. Ventilation, diffusion, and pefusion (718)
43. Zone I—a very small part of the apex
    Zone II—above the level of the left atrium
    Zone III—lung bases (732-733)
44. A shift in the oxyhemoglobin dissociation curve by changes in carbon dioxide and hydrogen ion concentrations in the blood (736)
45. Respiratory bronchioles, alveolar ducts, and alveoli (721)

Alterations of Pulmonary Function

Name _____

True/False

1. (T,743)   1. T   F   Respiratory alteration is the most common cause of hypoxemia.

2. (F,748)   2. T   F   If a pleural effusion is impairing pulmonary function, thoracentesis may be per
                         formed to drain the fluid away, the maximum amount of fluid being approximately
                         20 milliliters.

3. (F,750)   3. T   F   Pneumoconiosis is a pneumonia caused by pneumococci.

4. (T,741)   4. T   F   Dyspnea is an objectively observable condition.

5. (F,754)   5. T   F   Morbidity and mortality for asthma is declining.

6. (F,758)   6. T   F   Persons with an α_1-antitrypsin deficiency are predisposed to asthma.

7. (T,761)   7. T   F   Tuberculosis is transmitted from person to person through airborne droplets.

8. (F,763)   8. T   F   A pulmonary artery pressure of 23 mm Hg represents a normal state.

9. (T,764)   9. T   F   Chronic pulmonary hypertension can lead to cor pulmonale.

10. (T,766)   10. T   F   Lung cancer is the most frequent cause of cancer death in the United States.

11. (F,768)   11. T   F   Adenocarcinoma, a type of lung cancer, shows late metastasis.

Multiple Choice

12. (b,741)   12. _____ is generally relieved by sitting up in a forward leaning posture.

    a.   Dyspnea on exertion
    b.   Orthopnea
    c.   Apnea
    d.   Tachypnea

13. (b,741)   13. Kussmaul respiration may be characterized as:

    a.   alternating periods of deep and shallow breathing.
    b.   slightly increased ventilatory rate, large tidal volumes, and no expiratory pause.
    c.   the result of chronic obstructive pulmonary disease.
    d.   the result of pulmonary fibrosis.

14. (a,741) | 14. _____ are characterized by alternating periods of deep and shallow breathing.

   a. Cheyne-Stokes respirations
   b. Frank-Starling respirations
   c. Apnea respirations
   d. Orthopnea respirations

15. (c,741) | 15. Which of the following is a true statement?

   a. Hypoventilation causes hypocapnia.
   b. Hyperventilation causes hypercapnia.
   c. Hyperventilation causes hypocapnea.
   d. Hyperventilation results in an increased $PaCO_2$.

16. (a,741) | 16. Hypocapnia may be a result of:

   a. hyperventilation.
   b. hypoventilation.
   c. apnea.
   d. cyanosis.

17. (b,742) | 17. _____ is the selective bulbous enlargement of the distal segment of a digit and is commonly associated with diseases that interfere with oxygenation of the blood.

   a. Cyanosis
   b. Clubbing
   c. Angling
   d. Bullae

18. (c,743) | 18. _____ is reduced oxygenation of arterial blood caused by respiratory alterations.

   a. Ischemia
   b. Hypoxia
   c. Hypoxemia
   d. Hypocapnia

19. (a,743) | 19. _____ may result in hypoxemia.

   a. Hypoventilation
   b. Decreased nitrogen content of inspired gas
   c. Increased nitrogen content of inspired gas
   d. Left-to-right shunt
   e. Hyperpnea

20. (c,743) | 20. High altitudes may produce hypoxemia through:

   a. shunting.
   b. hypoventilation.
   c. decreased inspired oxygen.
   d. diffusion abnormalities.

21. (e,745) | 21. Pulmonary edema may be caused by:

   a. abnormal capillary hydrostatic pressure.
   b. abnormal capillary oncotic pressure.
   c. abnormal capillary permeability.
   d. both a and c
   e. a, b, and c

22. (b,745)   22. The most common cause of pulmonary edema is:

   a. right-sided heart failure.
   b. left-sided heart failure.
   c. mitral valve prolapse.
   d. aortic stenosis.

23. (b,745)   23. Clinical manifestations of severe pulmonary edema include:

   a. unlabored respirations.
   b. pink, frothy sputum.
   c. hypocapnia.
   d. anoxia.

24. (c,746)   24. _____ is the collapse of lung tissue due to the removal of air from obstructed or hypoventilated alveoli.

   a. Compression atelectasis
   b. Perfusion atelectasis
   c. Absorption atelectasis
   d. Hypoventilation atelectasis

25. (c,746)   25. In _____ bronchiectasis, constrictions and dilatations deform the bronchi.

   a. cylindrical
   b. symmetrical
   c. varicose
   d. saccular

26. (c,748)   26. In _____ pleural effusion the fluid is watery and diffuses out of the capillaries as a result of increased blood pressure or decreased capillary oncotic pressure.

   a. exudative
   b. purulent
   c. transudative
   d. infected

27. (b,748)   27. _____ is an infected pleural effusion, the presence of pus in the pleural space, and a complication of respiratory infection, usually pneumonia.

   a. Transudative effusion
   b. Empyema
   c. Exudative effusion
   d. Chyle

28. (c,749)   28. _____ is a circumscribed area of suppuration and destruction of lung parenchyma.

   a. A consolidation
   b. A cavitation
   c. An abscess
   d. A pleurisy

29. (d,750)   29. Inhalation of _____ is a cause for pneumoconiosis.

   a. silica
   b. asbestos
   c. mica
   d. all of the above

30. (b,751-752)   30. Which of the following shows a correct sequence in acute (adult) respiratory distress syndrome?

    a.   impaired alveolar compliance and recoil, causing decreased surfactant production
    b.   alveolocapillary membrane injury, causing damage to the surfactant producing alveoli
    c.   hyaline membrane formation and fibrosis, causing pulmonary edema
    d.   increased alveolocapillary membrane permeability, causing decreased surfactant production

31. (a,750)   31. _____ is a fulminant form of respiratory failure characterized by acute lung inflammation and diffuse alveolocapillary injury.

    a.   Acute (adult) respiratory distress syndrome
    b.   Sarcoidosis
    c.   Postoperative respiratory failure
    d.   Malignant respiratory failure

32. (b,752-753)   32. In _____ pulmonary disease either more force is required to expire a given volume of air or emptying of the lungs is slowed or both.

    a.   restrictive
    b.   obstructive
    c.   atelectic
    d.   acute atelectic

33. (c,754)   33. Asthma is thought to be caused by:

    a.   genetic inheritance.
    b.   environmental factors.
    c.   both a and b.
    d.   neither a nor b.

34. (d,755)   34. _____ asthma is characterized by continual symptoms, limited physical activity, and frequent exacerbations.

    a.   Step 1
    b.   Step 2
    c.   Step 3
    d.   Step 4

35. (e,754)   35. Asthma is classified by:

    a.   severity of symptoms.
    b.   degree of activity limitation.
    c.   pulmonary function tests.
    d.   number of emergency or hospital visits.
    e.   all of the above.

36. (a,756)   36. In chronic bronchitis _____ may lead to closure of the airway, particularly during expiration, when the airways are narrowed.

    a.   thick mucus from hypertrophied glands
    b.   infection
    c.   hyperventilation
    d.   thinning smooth muscle in the bronchioles

37. (b,756)   37. Emphysema differs from chronic bronchitis in that:

a. emphysema obstruction results from mucus production and inflammation.
b. emphysema obstruction results from changes in lung tissues.
c. chronic bronchitis obstruction results from changes in lung tissues.
d. there are no visual differences between the two conditions.

38. (c,756)   38. _____ is an abnormal permanent enlargement of gas exchange airways accompanied by destruction of alveolar walls.

a. COPD
b. Asthma
c. Emphysema
d. Adult respiratory distress syndrome

39. (c,757)   39. Individuals with a recent diagnosis of emphysema most often present with:

a. a productive cough.
b. cyanosis.
c. dyspnea.
d. cor pulmonale.

40. (a,761)   40. Which of the following is not one of the four phases of the inflammatory response associated with pneumococcal pneumonia?

a. atelectasis
b. consolidation
c. resolution
d. red hepatization

41. (e,763)   41. A massive pulmonary embolism may lead to:

a. shock.
b. hypotension.
c. pulmonary hypertension.
d. tachypnea.
e. all of the above.

42. (e,762)   42. Pulmonary embolism is occlusion of a portion of the pulmonary vascular bed by an embolus of:

a. fat.
b. air.
c. tissue fragment.
d. blood clot.
e. any of the above.

43. (a,763)   43. Pulmonary hypertension is defined as a rise in pulmonary artery pressure (normally 15 to 18 mm of Hg) of _____ mm Hg above normal.

a. 5 to 10
b. 10 to 15
c. 15 to 20
d. 20 to 25

44. (e,764) | 44. Cor pulmonale is:

    a. pulmonary heart disease.
    b. right ventricular enlargement.
    c. right ventricular dilatation.
    d. secondary to pulmonary hypertension.
    e. all of the above.

Matching

45. (d,745) | 45. ____ aspiration   a. accumulation of air in pleural space

46. (g,746) | 46. ____ compression atelectasis   b. inflammation of the pleura

47. (j,746) | 47. ____ bronchiectasis   c. the result of rib or sternal fractures

48. (a,747) | 48. ____ pneumothorax   d. the passage of fluid and solid particles into the lung

49. (i,748) | 49. ____ pleural effusion   e. inflammatory obstruction of small airways

50. (h,748) | 50. ____ empyema   f. excessive amount of connective tissue in the lung

51. (b,749) | 51. ____ pleurisy   g. alveolar collapse

52. (f,749) | 52. ____ pulmonary fibrosis   h. pus in the pleural space

53. (c,749) | 53. ____ flail chest   i. accumulation of fluid in the pleural space

54. (e,746) | 54. ____ bronchiolitis   j. abnormal dilation of the bronchi

Short Answer

55. What is the average respiratory rate range?

56. What is the average tidal volume range?

57. When will Kussmaul respiration be seen?

58. What are the characteristics of hemoptysis and hematemesis?

59. What other types of pain mimic pleuritic chest pain?

60. List four causes of hypercapnia.

61. What is the most common cause of hypoxemia?

62. Define acute respiratory failure.

63. What is the most common cause of pulmonary edema?

64. Why is the right lung more susceptible to aspiration than the left?

65. What type of pneumothorax is the most serious?

Short Answers

55. 8 to 16 breaths per minute (741)
56. 400 to 800 ml (741)
57. After strenuous exercise; in metabolic acidosis (741)
58. Hemoptysis: bright red; usually alkaline pH; mixed with frothy sputum
    Hematemesis: dark red; acid pH; mixed with food particles (742)
59. Cardiac pain, chest wall pain (742)
60. Drug-induced respiratory depression, diseases of the medulla, abnormalities in spinal nerve
    pathways, diseases of the neuromuscular junction, thoracic cage abnormalities, large airway
    obstruction, increased work of breathing or physiologic dead space (743)
61. Abnormal ventilation-perfusion ratio (743)
62. PaO_2 less than or equal to 50; $PaCO_2$ greater than or equal to 50; pH less than or equal to 7.25
    (744)
63. Heart disease (745)
64. The branching angle of the right main stem bronchus is straighter than the left (745-746)
65. Tension pneumothorax (747)

Alterations of Pulmonary Function in Children

Name _____

True/False

1. (T,782)   1.   T   F   The most common cause of bacterial pneumonia in children is *S. pneumoniae*.

2. (T,782)   2.   T   F   The most common cause of bacterial pneumonia in adolesents is *M. pneumoniae*.

3. (F,779)   3.   T   F   With treatment, less than 50% of infants with RDS survive.

4. (F,776)   4.   T   F   Epiglottitis is a mild, viral disease of children.

5. (T,784)   5.   T   F   Bronchopulmonary dysplasia can be cauused by oxygen toxicity.

6. (F,781)   6.   T   F   In asthma the older the child, the greater the risk for morbidity and mortality.

7. (T,779)   7.   T   F   Maternal diabetes can lead to respiratory distress in infants.

8. (T,779)   8.   T   F   The greatest single cause of death among infants between 1 week and 1 year of age is sudden infant death syndrome.

9. (T,779)   9.   T   F   RDS accounts for almost half of the deaths in the first year of life.

10. (T,779)   10. T   F   Asthma is the leading chronic illness in children.

11. (F,779)   11. T   F   Asthma-related death rates are lower in minority children.

Multiple Choice

12. (d,776)   12. The cause of 85% of croup cases is:

    a.   bacteria.
    b.   acute hyperventilation.
    c.   allergy.
    d.   viruses.

13. (c,778)   13. Which of the following types of croup is the most common?

    a.   acute epiglottitis.
    b.   viral croup.
    c.   acute laryngotracheobronchitis.
    d.   tracheitis.

14. Which of the following is a risk factor associated with sudden infant death syndrome?

a. preterm delivery
b. multiple pregnancies
c. low birth weight
d. a and b
e. a, b, and c

15. Risk factors associated with sudden infant death syndrome include all of the following *except*:

a. poor mothers younger than 20 years of age.
b. low birth weight.
c. smoking during pregnancy.
d. anemia during pregnancy.
e. frequent viral infections.

16. Sudden infant death syndrome occurs most often between _____ and _____ months of age.

a. 1, 3
b. 2, 3
c. 2, 4
d. 1, 4

17. _____ is (are) a sign of asthma.

a. edema of the bronchial mucosa
b. bronchospasms
c. mucous plugging of the airways
d. all of the above

18. About _____ % of asthmas in children is inherited.

a. 10
b. 20
c. 30
d. 40

19. With regard to an asthma attack, infants are at a disadvantage because of:

a. their relatively small alveolocapillary surface area.
b. increased resistance of their relatively narrow airways.
c. their mechanically disadvantaged diaphragm.
d. all of the above.

20. _____ is the most common cause of pneumonia in children.

a. Streptococcus pneumonia
b. Respiratory syncytial virus
c. *H. influenzae*
d. Staphylococcus pneumonia

21. Bronchiolitis, inflammatory obstruction of the bronchioles, tends to occur during the first two years of life, with a peak incidence at approximately _____ months of age.

a. 2
b. 4
c. 6
d. 8

22. (e,782)   22. _____ is an etiologic agent of childhood bronchiolitis.

    a. Respiratory syncitial virus
    b. Para influenza 3 virus
    c. Adenovirus
    d. Mycoplasma
    e. All of the above

23. (a,784)   23. _____ is a serious secondary disorder that has a high morbidity and mortality.

    a. Bronchiolitis obliterans
    b. Primary bronchiolitis
    c. Adenovirus-induced pneumonia
    d. Streptococcus-induced pneumonia

24. (c,779)   24. The chief predisposing factor for respiratory distress syndrome of the newborn is:

    a. low birth weight.
    b. alcohol consumption during pregnancy.
    c. premature birth.
    d. smoking during pregnancy.

25. (d,779)   25. Respiratory distress syndrome of the newborn is also called:

    a. hyaline membrane disease.
    b. idiopathic respiratory distress syndrome.
    c. surfactant respiratory distress syndrome.
    d. a and b
    e. all of the above

26. (a,781)   26. The primary predisposing factor of respiratory distress syndrome of the newborn is:

    a. premature birth.
    b. gender of the newborn.
    c. hypervolemia.
    d. hypovolemia.

27. (d,779)   27. The primary problem in respiratory distress of the newborn is:

    a. lack of surfactant.
    b. pulmonary edema.
    c. inadequate alveolar surface.
    d. a and c
    e. all of the above

28. (b,780)   28. Which of the following shows a correct sequence in respiratory distress syndrome of the new born?

    a. increased pulmonary vascular resistance, atelectasis, hypoperfusion
    b. hypoperfusion, hypoxic vasoconstriction, right-to-left shunt
    c. respiratory acidosis, hypoxemia, hypercapnia
    d. right-to-left shunt, hypoxic vasoconstriction, hypoperfusion

29. (a,784)

29. Cystic fibrosis can be characterized as:

    a. an autosomal recessive disease.
    b. an autosomal dominant disease.
    c. an X-linked recessive disease.
    d. an X-linked dominant disease.

30. (b,784)

30. Children with cystic fibrosis demonstrate elevated levels of which compound in both sweat and salivary gland secretions?

    a. potassium
    b. sodium chloride
    c. magnesium
    d. carbonic acid

31. (d,784)

31. _____ is an inherited disease of the exocrine glands resulting in the production of excessive, thick mucus that obstructs the gastrointestinal system and lungs.

    a. Cystic fibrosis
    b. Amyloidosis
    c. Mucoviscidosis
    d. a and c
    e. a, b, and c

Matching

32. (c, 783) 32. ___ viral pneumonia   a. *S. areus*

33. (b, 783) 33. ___ pneumococcal pneumonia   b. *S. pneumoniae*

34. (a, 783) 34. ___ staphylococcal pneumonia   c. RSV

35. (d, 783) 35. ___ streptococcal pneumonia   d. group A beta-hemolytic streptococci

Short Answer

36. What treatment is universal in children with epiglottitis?

37. List four risk factors for RDS.

38. What groups of children have higher morbidity and mortality from asthma?

39. In which seasons are viral infections more common in children?

40. What is the survival age for cystic fibrosis?

Short Answers

36. Intubation for 1 to 3 days (778)
37. Premature birth, male gender, cesarean delivery, diabetic mother, asphyxia, hypovolemia or hypervolemia, maternal antepartum hemorrhage, maternal shock (779)
38. Inner-city black and Hispanic children (779)
39. Winter and early spring with minor peaks in the fall (782)
40. About 30 years (785)

CHAPTER

28

Structure and Function of the Renal and Urologic Systems

Name _____

True/False

1. (T,793)

2. (T,795)

3. (F,794)

4. (T,795)

5. (F,790)

6. (F,797)

7. (F,797)

8. (T,798-799)

9. (T,799)

10. (F,799)

11. (F,802)

1. T F   The arcuate arteries branch to form the interlobar arteries.

2. T F   There is a direct relationship between renal blood flow and GFR.

3. T F   A ring of smooth muscle, the ureteral sphincter, surrounds the ureters where they enter the urinary bladder.

4. T F   Renal blood vessels are innervated by the autonomic nervous system.

5. T F   The kidneys are located in the posterior peritoneal cavity.

6. T F   Tubular secretion is the movements of fluids and solutes from the tubular lumen to the peritubular capillaries.

7. T F   Net filtration pressure involves only those forces which promote filtration.

8. T F   A urethral stricture may affect the glomerular filtration rate.

9. T F   Active transport in the renal tubules can be limited as the carrier molecules become saturated.

10. T F   The primary function of the proximal convoluted tubule is the secretion of sodium chloride.

11. T F   Generally, a diuretic increases the flow of urine through the direct stimulation of sodium reabsorption.

Multiple Choice

12. (e,790)

12. A medial indentation, the renal hilus, contains the entry and exit for the renal:

   a. blood vessels.
   b. nerves.
   c. lymphatic vessels.
   d. ureter.
   e. all of the above.

13. (b,791)

13. The area of the kidneys that contains the glomeruli of the nephrons is the:

    a. medulla.
    b. cortex.
    c. pyramids.
    d. columns.

14. (b,790)

14. The _____ is the functional unit of the kidney.

    a. glomerulus
    b. nephron
    c. collecting duct
    d. pyramid

15. (d,791)

15. All of the following are part of the nephron except the:

    a. loop of Henle.
    b. renal corpuscle.
    c. proximal convoluted tubule.
    d. calyx.

16. (b,791)

16. Which of the following is not a structure found in the kidney?

    a. pyramid
    b. adrenal cortex
    c. papilla
    d. major calyx

17. (b,791)

17. The nephrons that are the most important in determining the concentration of the urine are:

    a. the cortical nephrons.
    b. the juxtamedullary nephrons.
    c. a and b.
    d. neither a nor b.

18. (d,791)

18. Which of the following is a true statement regarding the glomerular filtration membrane?

    a. The layers are composed of podocytes.
    b. It allows for the filtration of blood cells.
    c. Proteins with a molecular weight of 80,000 can pass through the membrane.
    d. It is composed of three layers.

19. (c,791)

19. 85% of all nephrons are _____ nephrons.

    a. juxtamedullary
    b. juxtacortical
    c. cortical
    d. medullary

20. (a,791)

20. Together, the glomerulus and Bowman's capsule are referred to as:

    a. the renal corpuscle.
    b. the renal capsule.
    c. the renal medulla.
    d. the renal pyramid.
    e. the renal functional unit.

21. (d,793)

21. The _____ make up the juxtaglomerular apparatus.

    a. macula densa cells
    b. juxtaglomerular cells
    c. Bowman's capsule
    d. a and b
    e. a, b, and c

22. (b,793)

22. The renal structure that drains directly into the minor calyces is the:

    a. distal convoluted tubule.
    b. collecting duct.
    c. pyramid.
    d. renal pelvis.

23. (b,794)

23. The portion of the male urethra that is closest to the bladder is the:

    a. membranous.
    b. prostatic.
    c. cavernous.
    d. vas deferens.

24. (c,794)

24. The trigone may be defined as:

    a. the orifice of the ureter.
    b. the inner area of the kidney.
    c. a smooth triangular area between the openings of the two ureters and the urethra.
    d. the three divisions of the loop of Henle.

25. (a,797)

25. The filtration of the plasma per unit of time is known as the glomerular filtration rate (GFR). The GFR is directly related to the:

    a. perfusion pressure in the glomerular capillaries.
    b. diffusion rate in the renal cortex.
    c. diffusion rate in the renal medulla.
    d. glomerular active transport.

26. (c,795)

26. On average the kidneys receive approximately _____% to _____% of the cardiac output.

    a. 10, 20
    b. 15, 20
    c. 20, 25
    d. 30, 35

27. (a,795)

27. As systemic blood pressure falls, the afferent arterioles of the kidneys _____, preventing a reduction in blood flow to the glomerulus.

    a. dilate
    b. constrict
    c. neither; the efferent arteriole is the artery that autoregulates to keep the glomerular filtration rate constant

28. (d,796)

28. Renin, an enzyme secreted from the juxtaglomerular apparatus, causes the direct:

    a. activation of angiotensin I.
    b. activation of angiotensin II.
    c. release of ADH.
    d. activation of angiotensin I.

29. (b,795)

29. The blood vessels of the kidneys are innervated by the:

    a. vagus nerve.
    b. sympathetic nervous system.
    c. somatic nervous system.
    d. parasympathetic nervous system.

30. (c,795)

30. _____ is an enzyme that is synthesized and secreted by the juxtaglomerular apparatus.

    a. Angiotensin
    b. Angiotensinogen
    c. Renin
    d. Plasmin

31. (b,803)

31. Atrial natriuretic hormone eventually causes a(n) _____ in blood volume.

    a. increase
    b. decrease
    c. steady state

32. (c,795)

32. The kidney is a target tissue for all of the following *except*:

    a. aldosterone.
    b. atrial natriuretic hormone.
    c. angiotensin I.
    d. none of the above.

33. (d,793)

33. Which of the following is not an artery supplying the kidney?

    a. renal arteries
    b. interlobar arteries
    c. arcuate arteries
    d. hilar arteries

34. (b,797)

34. Which of the following structures of the nephron is not involved in the secretion of hydrogen ions?

    a. proximal tubule
    b. loop of Henle
    c. distal tubule
    d. collecting duct

35. (d,800)

35. The descending loop of the nephron primarily allows for:

    a. sodium secretion.
    b. potassium secretion.
    c. hydrogen ion secretion.
    d. water reabsorption.

36. (a,801)

36. The concentration of the final urine is determined by antidiuretic hormone (ADH), which is secreted by the:

    a. posterior pituitary.
    b. right atrium.
    c. left atrium.
    d. thalamus.

37. (c,803)   37. _____ is (are) a hormone synthesized and secreted by the kidneys.

a. Antidiuretic hormone
b. Aldosterone
c. Erythropoietin
d. Angiotensinogen
e. All of the above

38. (a,803)   38. The best estimate of functioning renal tissue is:

a. GFR.
b. circulating ADH levels.
c. volume of urine output.
d. the specific gravity of the solute concentration of the urine.

39. (a,804)   39. Blood urea nitrogen (BUN) levels _____ as glomerular filtration decreases.

a. increase
b. decrease
c. remain unchanged because urea is not retained by the glomerulus

40. (d,802)   40. Oliguria is defined as a 24-hour urine output of less than:

a. 1000 ml.
b. 800 ml.
c. 500 ml.
d. 400 ml.

41. (c,803)   41. GFR and plasma creatinine concentration are _____ related.

a. directly
b. indirectly
c. inversely
d. not

Ordering

42.   42. Trace filtrate through the nephron by numbering the following in correct order.

(3,791)   ____   descending limb

(7,791)   ____   collecting duct

(1,791)   ____   glomerulus

(6,791)   ____   distal convoluted tubule

(4,791)   ____   loop of Henle

(5,791)   ____   ascending limb

(2,791)   ____   proximal convoluted tubule

Short Answer

43. Name the two types of nephrons.

44. Name the three layers of the glomular filtration membrane.

45. Where are the kidneys located?

46. Which kidney is lower? Why?

47. List the four functions of the nephron.

48. What is the total volume of fluid filtered by the glomeruli daily? What percentage is reabsorbed?

49. List two changes in renal function that occur with aging?

Short Answers

43. Cortical and juxtamedullary (791)
44. Inner capillary endothelium, middle basement membrane, outer capillary epithelium (791)
45. Retroperitonally, on either side of the vertebral column from the twelfth thoracic to the third lumbar vertebra (790)
46. The right kidney is slightly lower because it is displaced downward by the liver. (790)
47. (1) Filters plasma at the glomerulus; (2) reabsorbs and secretes different substances along tubular structure; (3) forms filtrate of protein-free plasma; (4) regulates the filtrate to maintain body fluid volume, electrolyte composition, and pH within narrow limits (796)
48. 180 L/day; 99% (798, 800)
49. Number of nephrons decreases; degenerative changes decrease ability to concentrate urine or tolerate fluctuations in fluid balance; delayed response to pH change; delayed ability to reabsorb glucose; decreased ability to eliminate drugs; alterations in thirst may alter water balance; impairment in renal function, hormone regulatory systems, and medication use may alter sodium and water balance. (805)

Alterations of Renal and Urinary Tract Function

Name _____

True/False

1. (T,808)	1. T	F	Postobstructive diuresis often occurs after a urinary tract obstruction is removed.
2. (T,808)	2. T	F	Complications of urinary obstruction include a reduction in glomerular filtration rate.
3. (T,808)	3. T	F	Urinary tract obstruction can lead to renal failure.
4. (T,810)	4. T	F	A neurogenic bladder is a functional urinary tract obstruction caused by an interruption of the nerve supply to the bladder.
5. (F,811)	5. T	F	The most common type of renal neoplasm is a renal adenoma.
6. (T,812)	6. T	F	Women with bacteriuria may be asymptomatic.
7. (F,812)	7. T	F	Urinary tract infections are usually caused by viruses.
8. (F,818)	8. T	F	Two clinical manifestations of nephrotic syndrome include decreased glomerular permeability to and increased proximal tubule reabsorption of protein.
9. (F,819)	9. T	F	Azotemia is associated with a decrease in serum urea levels.
10. (T,821-822)	10. T	F	Potassium is usually retained in chronic renal failure and requires dietary restriction.
11. (F,822)	11. T	F	Chronic renal failure can be diagnosed only by renal biopsy.
12. (F,822)	12. T	F	The major treatment for end-stage renal failure is diuretics.
13. (F,819)	13. T	F	Symptoms of end-stage renal failure develop when 50% of kidney function is lost.
14. (T,822)	14. T	F	Nutrition management is essential for a patient with chronic renal failure.

Multiple Choice

15. (e,808)

15. The pathophysiologic consequences of urinary tract obstruction are related to:

    a. location of the obstruction.
    b. unilateral or bilateral involvement.
    c. partial or complete obstruction.
    d. acute or chronic obstruction.
    e. all of the above.

16. (c,809)

16. The most common type of renal stone is:

    a. magnesium.
    b. struvite.
    c. calcium.
    d. phosphate.

17. (b,809)

17. Staghorn calculi grow in the _____ of the kidney and have the shape of a stag's horns.

    a. renal pelvis only
    b. renal pelvis and into the calyces
    c. renal pelvis and into the ureters
    d. none of the above; calculi never grow to such an extent

18. (e,812)

18. Which of the following organisms is known to cause cystitis?

    a. *Proteus*
    b. *Escherichia coli*
    c. *Klebsiella*
    d. b and c
    e. a, b, and c

19. (a,812)

19. About_____% of individuals with bacteriuria have no symptoms, and_____% of individuals with symptoms have no bacteriuria.

    a. 10, 30
    b. 20, 40
    c. 30, 10
    d. 40, 20

20. (d,812)

20. One of the most common infecting organisms of the urinary tract is:

    a. adenovirus.
    b. herpes virus.
    c. pox virus.
    d. *E. coli.*

21. (a,813)

21. Pyelonephritis, an infection of the renal pelvis and interstitium, is usually caused by:

    a. bacteria.
    b. fungi.
    c. viruses.
    d. b and c.
    e. all of the above.

22. (b,813)

22. Which of the following is not a cause of pyelonephritis?

    a.   pregnancy
    b.   glomerulonephritis
    c.   kidney stones
    d.   neurogenic bladder

23. (c,815)

23. A patient is demonstrating hematuria with red blood cell casts and proteinuria exceeding 3 to 5 g/day, with albumin as the major protein. The most probable diagnosis is:

    a.   cystitis.
    b.   chronic pyelonephritis.
    c.   glomerulonephritis.
    d.   nephrotic syndrome.

24. (c,815)

24. Acute glomerulonephritis is usually associated with:

    a.   *E. coli.*
    b.   herpes vírus.
    c.   streptococcus (postinfection).
    d.   none of the above.

25. (a,815)

25. Goodpasture syndrome is an example of:

    a.   rapidly progressive glomerulonephritis.
    b.   chronic glomerulonephritis.
    c.   chronic pyelonephritis.
    d.   acute pyelonephritis.

26. (c,815)

26. In the treatment of rapidly progressive glomerulonephritis, plasmapheresis is usually combined with prednisone and cyclophosphamide to suppress a rebound:

    a.   infection.
    b.   in virus replication.
    c.   in antibody formation.
    d.   antidiuretic hormone production.

27. (c,816)

27. _____ is an immune mechanism that commonly contributes to glomerulonephritis.

    a.   Deposition of circulating soluble antigen-antibody complexes into the glomueruli
    b.   Formation of antibodies against the glomerular basement membrane
    c.   Both a and b
    d.   None of the above

28. (e,818)

28. The pathophysiology of nephrotic syndrome is primarily related to:

    a.   an injured glomerular filtration membrane.
    b.   loss of plasma proteins.
    c.   loss of albumin and several immunoglobulins.
    d.   b and c.
    e.   a, b, and c.

29. (a,819)

29. Hypovolemia may cause which of the following types of acute renal failures?

    a.   prerenal
    b.   intrarenal
    c.   postrenal
    d.   transrenal

30. (e,819)

30. _____ may cause prerenal acute renal failure.

   a. Hypotension
   b. Hypovolemia
   c. Cardiac insufficiency
   d. a and b
   e. a, b, and c

31. (c,821)

31. Which of the following statements concerning chronic renal failure is not true?

   a. Plasma creatinine level increases.
   b. Sodium excretion increases.
   c. Alkalosis develops.
   d. Potassium is retained.

32. (c,822)

32. In chronic renal failure, _____ are restricted in the diet.

   a. fats
   b. carbohydrates
   c. proteins
   d. a and b
   e. a, b, and c

33. (c,823)

33. Anemia accompanies chronic renal failure because of:

   a. blood loss via the urine.
   b. renal insensitivity to vitamin D.
   c. inadequate production of erythropoietin.
   d. inadequate retention of serum iron.

34. (b,823)

34. Pruritus, seen in patients with end-stage renal disease, is due to high levels of:

   a. potassium.
   b. calcium.
   c. sodium.
   d. magnesium.

35. (c,823)

35. Anemia of renal failure can be successfully treated with:

   a. intrinsic factor.
   b. vitamin B.
   c. recombinant human erythropoietin.
   d. iron.

Matching

36. (b,813)

36. ____ pyelonephritis

a. inflammation of the bladder

37. (d,815)

37. ____ rapidly progressing glomerulonephritis

b. infection of the renal pelvis and interstitium

38. (a,812)

38. ____ cystitis

c. occurs afer streptococcal infection

39. (e,815)

39. ____ excessive proteinuria

d. Goodpasture syndrome

40. (c,815)

40. ____ acute glomerulonephritis

e. nephrotic syndrome

Short Answer

41. Renal insufficiency occurs when _____ % of function is lost.

42. What are the three types of acute renal failure?

43. What are the three major kinds of renal stones?

44. What is the hallmark symptom of a renal stone?

45. List four common causes of pyelonephritis.

Short Answers

41. About 75% (818)
42. Prerenal, intrarenal, and postrenal (819)
43. Calcium, struvite, uric acid (809)
44. Pain (801)
45. Kidney stones, vesicoureteral reflux, pregnancy, neurogenic bladder, instrumentation, female sexual trauma (813)

Alterations of Renal and Urinary Function in Children

Name _____

True/False

1. (F,828)   1. T   F   Abnormal urinary tract anatomy is seen in only 5% of the total population.

2. (T,828)   2. T   F   Renal disease may be hereditary.

3. (T,828)   3. T   F   Almost half of all children with renal failure have structural abnormalities in the renal system.

4. (F,828)   4. T   F   Down syndrome is frequently associated with urinary tract malformations.

5. (T,828)   5. T   F   Approximately one-third of the people with horseshoe kidneys are asymptomatic.

6. (T,828)   6. T   F   Chordee is a congenital defect of the genitourinary tract that results in a ventral curvature of the penis.

7. (F,829)   7. T   F   Epispadias may be found only in males.

8. (T,829)   8. T   F   Exstrophy of the bladder is a congenital anomaly in which the lower urinary tract is exposed directly to the surface of the body.

9. (T,829)   9. T   F   Unilateral renal agenesis is the total lack of one kidney and happens more often on the left side and in males.

10. (F,829)   10. T   F   Renal agenesis is always clearly hereditary.

11. (T,830)   11. T   F   Over 50% of renal failure in children is due to chronic glomerulonephritis.

12. (T,831)   12. T   F   Hemolytic uremic syndrome frequently causes acute renal failure in children.

13. (F,832)   13. T   F   Vesicoureteral reflux is always bilateral.

14. (T,833)   14. T   F   Wilms tumor is an embryonal tumor of the kidney.

15. (F,834)   15. T   F   Secondary enuresis refers to a condition in which the child has never been continent.

16. (F,834)   16. T   F   Organic causes of enuresis are the most common.

Multiple Choice

17. (c,833)   17. Wilms tumor:

    a. is usually symptomatic when diagnosed.
    b. causes flank swelling.
    c. is usually encapsulated.
    d. has a peak incidence between 4-5 years.

18. (a,832)   18. Vesicoureteral reflux:
    a. may be hereditary.
    b. is more common in boys.
    c. occurs most often in black children.
    d. is rarely seen with UTI.

19. (b,831)   19. Children with IgA nephropathy have recurrent:

    a. infections.
    b. hematuria.
    c. vomiting.
    d. enuresis.

20. (d,831)   20. In children, the most common cause of acute renal failure is:

    a. infection.
    b. obstruction.
    c. nephrotic syndrome.
    d. hemolytic uremic syndrome.

21. (a,829)   21. A common cause of chronic renal failure in children is:

    a. bilateral hypoplastic kidney.
    b. renal agenesis.
    c. hemolytic uremic syndrome.
    d. vesicoureteral reflux.

22. (d,828)   22. The most common problems associated with horseshoe kidneys include:

    a. hydronephrosis.
    b. infection.
    c. stone formation.
    d. all of the above.

23. (a,828)   23. Upon examination of a child, it is determined that the urethral meatus is located on the under
        surface of the penis. This condition is called:

    a. hypospadias.
    b. epispadias.
    c. hydroureter.
    d. nidus.

24. (d,829)   24. Which of the following statements concerning renal agenesis is not correct?

    a. Bilateral renal agenesis occurs more often in males.
    b. Unilateral renal agenesis occurs more often than bilateral renal agenesis.
    c. Bilateral renal agenesis is also called Potter syndrome.
    d. Renal agenesis is not congenital.

25. (e,829)

25. Bilateral renal agenesis is often associated with:

   a.   parrot-beak nose.
   b.   wide-set eyes.
   c.   low-set ears.
   d.   a and c.
   e.   a, b, and c.

26. (c,829)

26. Forty percent of infants who have bilateral renal agenesis:

   a.   die within one year of birth.
   b.   die within one day of birth.
   c.   are stillborn.
   d.   live until puberty.

27. (b,830)

27. Which of the following is not considered part of the nephrotic syndrome in children?

   a.   proteinuria
   b.   decreased BUN
   c.   hyperlipidemia
   d.   lipiduria

28. (e,830)

28. Which of the following is indicative of nephrotic syndrome?

   a.   proteinuria
   b.   hyperlipidemia
   c.   lipiduria
   d.   a and c
   e.   a, b, and c

29. (b,830)

29. If nephrotic syndrome is not caused initially by kidney failure, it is termed _____ nephrotic syndrome.

   a.   primary
   b.   secondary
   c.   tertiary
   d.   idiopathic

30. (c,830)

30. One of the indications of nephrotic syndrome in children is:

   a.   sunken fontanelles.
   b.   pretibial edema.
   c.   frothy urine.
   d.   jaundice.

31. (d,830)

31. Poststreptococcal glomerulonephritis may be a sequela to:

   a.   varicella sores.
   b.   pharyngeal infections.
   c.   infected insect bites.
   d.   all of the above.

32. (a,831)

32. Urinary tract infections are uncommon in newborns, and when they occur they are usually:

   a.   blood-borne infections.
   b.   caused by bacteria from the GI tract.
   c.   yeast infections.
   d.   viral infections.

33. (a,832)   33. _____ is the retrograde flow of urine from the urinary bladder into the ureters.

 a. Vesicoureteral reflux
 b. Vesicourethral reflux
 c. Vesicourethral influx
 d. Hydronephrosis

34. (b,833)   34. _____ is often associated with Wilms tumor.

 a. Renal anaplasia
 b. Aniridia (lack of an iris in the eye)
 c. Anemia
 d. Hypothyroidism

35. (e,833)   35. Congenital anomalies seen with Wilms tumor include:

 a. polycystic kidneys.
 b. aniridia.
 c. hemihypertrophy.
 d. a and c.
 e. a, b, and c.

Matching

36. (d,834)   36. ___ total incontinence   a. sudden uncontrollable need to void

37. (f,834)   37. ___ overflow incontinence   b. incontinence in spite of normal voiding

38. (a,834)   38. ___ urge incontinence   c. voiding while laughing or coughing

39. (e,834)   39. ___ precipitate voiding   d. inability to store any urine

40. (c,834)   40. ___ stress incontinence   e. voiding without urge

41. (b,834)   41. ___ paradoxic incontinence   f. frequent dribbling

Short Answer

42. Bladder control is usually accomplished by age _____.

43. Prune-belly syndrome indicates what anomoly?

44. What is the most common form of glomerulonephritis worldwide?

45. The peak incidence for Wilms tumor occurs between ages _____ and _____.

Short Answers

42. 4 years (834)
43. Renal dysplasia (829)
44. IgA nephropathy (831)
45. 2 and 3 years (833)

CHAPTER

31

Structure and Function of the Reproductive Systems

Name _____

True/False

1. (T, 838)

1. T   F   The male and female genital organs are homologous before eight weeks of gestation.

2. (F,840)

2. T   F   Production of sperm begins during fetal life.

3. (T,843)

3. T   F   The uterus plays an important role in the sexual response.

4. (T,843)

4. T   F   At puberty the uterus descends from the abdomen to the lower pelvis.

5. (T,847)

5. T   F   The structure of the vagina undergoes cyclic changes with the menstrual cycle.

6. (T,847)

6. T   F   During the luteal/secretory phase of the menstrual cycle, estrogen levels begin to dip and progesterone levels begin to rise.

7. (F,847)

7. T   F   At the breasts, progesterone acts to increase the actions of prolactin.

8. (F,854)

8. T   F   The primary spermatocyte has a total of 23 chromosomes.

Multiple Choice

9. (b,838)

9. Until the _____ week of gestation, the initial reproductive structures of the male and female appear the same.

   a.   third
   b.   eighth
   c.   twentieth
   d.   thirtieth

10. (d,839)

10. The major hormonal determinant of sexual differentiation in utero is:

   a.   estrogen.
   b.   progesterone.
   c.   growth hormone.
   d.   testosterone.

11. (e, 840)

11. Hormonal stimulation of the reproductive system involves the:

 a. gonads.
 b. central nervous system.
 c. endocrine system.
 d. hypothalamus.
 e. all of the above.

12. (c,840)

12. Which of the following shows a correct sequence in the hormonal stimulation of the reproductive systems leading to puberty?

 a. anterior pituitary, GnRH, FSH and LH
 b. hypothalamus, FSH, anterior pituitary
 c. anterior pituitary, FSH and LH, gonads
 d. GnRH, hypothalamus, FSH and LH

13. (a,841)

13. All of the following are classified as external female genitalia except the:

 a. vagina.
 b. labia majora.
 c. clitoris.
 d. vestibule.
 e. labia minora.

14. (c,843)

14. The thick middle layer of the uterine wall is the:

 a. epithelial layer.
 b. endometrium.
 c. myometrium.
 d. perimetrium.

15. (b,843)

15. The _____ is lined with columnar epithelial cells.

 a. perimetrium
 b. endocervical canal
 c. myometrium
 d. vagina

16. (c,844)

16. The usual site of fertilization is the:

 a. uterus.
 b. fimbriae.
 c. ampulla of the fallopian tubes.
 d. os of the fallopian tubes.

17. (a,845)

17. Sex hormones are secreted by the following cells in the ovary, except the _____ cells.

 a. endothelial
 b. stromal
 c. thecal
 d. granulosa
 e. corpus luteum

18. (d,845) | 18. Cells of the ovary that secrete hormones have receptors for:

   a. gonadotropins.
   b. FSH.
   c. LH.
   d. all of the above.

19. (c,847) | 19. Having ejected a mature ovum, the ovarian follicle develops into:

   a. an atretic follicle.
   b. a thecal follicle.
   c. a corpus luteum.
   d. a scar.

20. (a,845) | 20. The most potent of the following estrogens is:

   a. estradiol.
   b. testosterone.
   c. estrone.
   d. estriol.

21. (b,845) | 21. Which of the following is a true statement?

   a. Testosterone production is absent in the normal female.
   b. The precursor for the sex hormones is cholesterol.
   c. Estriol is the most potent type of estrogen.
   d. Granulosa cells act independently to produce ovarian estrogen.

22. (e,845) | 22. Estrogen has metabolic effects on the:

   a. endometrium.
   b. liver.
   c. blood vessels.
   d. bones.
   e. all of the above.

23. (c,840) | 23. _____ induces gonadotrophin synthesis by the anterior pituitary.

   a. FSH
   b. LH
   c. GnRH
   d. None of the above
   e. All of the above

24. (d,846) | 24. Progesterone is often referred to as "the hormone of pregnancy." Which of the following represents its action during pregnancy?

   a. stimulation of lactation during fetal development
   b. increased motility and ciliary action in the fallopian tubes
   c. thinning of the myometrium
   d. maintenance of the thickened endometrium

25. (a,847) | 25. Menstruation is followed by the _____ phase of the menstrual cycle.

   a. follicular
   b. luteal
   c. secretory
   d. none of the above

26. (b,848)

26. During the menstrual cycle, ovulation occurs following:

    a.   the gradual decrease in estrogen levels.
    b.   the surge of LH.
    c.   the sharp rise in progesterone.
    d.   b and c.
    e.   a, b, and c.

27. (d,848)

27. To grow and mature, ovarian follicles require:

    a.   FSH.
    b.   LH.
    c.   ACTH.
    d.   a and b.
    e.   all of the above.

28. (b,848)

28. The LH surge transforms granulosa cells into:

    a.   thecal cells.
    b.   corpus luteal cells.
    c.   scars.
    d.   fibroblasts.

29. (e,849)

29. _____ promotes the formation of channels in the mucus of the cervical os, providing channels for sperm.

    a.   LH
    b.   FSH
    c.   Testosterone
    d.   Estrogen
    e.   Progesterone

30. (e,850)

30. The functions of the testes include:

    a.   production of androgens.
    b.   production of gametes.
    c.   production of gonadotropins.
    d.   a and b.
    e.   a, b, and c.

31. (c,850)

31. Spermatogenesis occurs in the:

    a.   epididymis.
    b.   testes.
    c.   seminiferous tubules.
    d.   vas deferens.

32. (a,853)

32. _____ are a pair of glands that lie posterior to the urinary bladder in the male.

    a.   Seminal vesicles
    b.   Prostate glands
    c.   Cowper's glands
    d.   Parabladder glands

33. (e,852-853)   33. Which of the following contribute to the ejaculate?

a. prostate gland
b. seminal vesicles
c. Cowper's glands
d. a and b
e. a, b, and c

34. (a,851)   34. The internal genitalia of the male includes all of the following except the:

a. epididymidis.
b. vas deferens.
c. prostate gland.
d. seminal vesicles.
e. Cowper's glands.

35. (b,855)   35. The major difference between male and female sex hormone production is that:

a. LH has no apparent action in the male.
b. in the male, sex hormone production is relatively constant.
c. estradiol is not produced in the male.
d. in the male, GnRH does not cause the release of FSH.

36. (b,855)   36. The glands of Montgomery are located in the:

a. testes.
b. breasts.
c. uterus.
d. vagina.

37. (e,856)   37 Which of the following hormones plays a role in female breast development?

a. cortisol
b. prolactin
c. thyroid hormone
d. a and b
e. a, b, and c

38. (c,857)   38. Which of the following is not a characteristic associated with declining ovarian function with age?

a. vasomotor flush
b. decline in bone mass
c. postmenopausal decreased risk of coronary disease
d. atrophy of the uterus

39. (a,858)   39. Which of the following is not a normal characteristic of aging and the male reproductive system?

a. shortened refractory time
b. changes in libido
c. testicular atrophy
d. a and b
e. a, b, and c

Matching

40. (849)	40. ___ follicle develops; endometrium proliferates	a. early follicular phase
		b. late follicular phase
41. (849)	41. ___ menstruation begins	
		c. ovulatory phase
42. (849)	42. ___ functional layer of endometrium is shed	d. early luteal phase
43. (849)	43. ___ surge of GnRH, FSH, and LH	e. late luteal phase
44. (849)	44. ___ corpus luteum begins to develop	f. menstrual phase
45. (849)	45. ___ endometrium ready for implantation	

Short Answer

46. Puberty begins about age _____ for boys and about age _____ for girls.

47. What two factors enable the vagina to be self-cleaning and resist infection?

48. List two abnormalities that can cause estrogen disturbances.

49. How long does the process of spermatogenesis take?

Short Answers

46. 11, 10 (839)
47. The acid-base balance; the thickness of the vaginal epithelium (843)
48. Abnormalities in secretion of GnRH by the hypothalamus, secretion of LH or FSH by the anterior pituitary, hormonal feedback mechanisms, or structural integrity of the ovaries. (845)
49. 70 to 80 days (854)

Alterations of the Reproductive Systems

Including Sexually Transmitted Infections

Name _____

True/False

1. (T,862) 1. T F Delay of puberty seldom requires treatment, unless the delay is causing psycho-social problems.

2. (F,863) 2. T F Primary amenorrhea is normal during early adolesence, pregnancy, and lactation and when menopause is approaching.

3. (T,863) 3. T F Genetic disorders may result in amenorrhea.

4. (F,865) 4. T F A predisposition to premenstrual syndrome is clearly genetic.

5. (T,866) 5. T F Infection of the fallopian tubes is termed salpingitis.

6. (T,874) 6. T F In a person with endometriosis, endometrial tissue that responds to hormonal changes of the menstrual cycle may be found in the lungs.

7. (T,875) 7. T F Cervical cancer is generally considered a sexually transmitted disease.

8. (T,876) 8. T F With early diagnosis and treatment of cervical cancer, prognosis is excellent.

9. (T,886) 9. T F Testicular tumors are slightly more common on the right side than on the left.

Multiple Choice

10. (c,862) 10. In 90% to 95% of cases of delayed puberty the problem is:

    a.   because of a disruption in the hypothalamus.
    b.   because of a disruption of the pituitary.
    c.   slow maturation.
    d.   decreased hormone levels.

11. (b,862)

11. A female patient, age 6, is showing growth of pubic hair. All other physical characteristics appear normal. The correct diagnosis would be:

   a.   delayed puberty.
   b.   incomplete precocious puberty.
   c.   heterosexual precocious puberty.
   d.   normal puberty.

12. (a,862)

12. _____ causes the child to develop some secondary sex characteristics of the opposite sex.

   a.   Heterosexual precocious puberty
   b.   Incomplete precocious puberty
   c.   Isosexual precocious puberty
   d.   Homosexual precocious puberty

13. (d,863)

13. All of the following may be causes of primary amenorrhea *except*:

   a.   the hypothalamus dysfunctions.
   b.   the pituitary dysfunctions.
   c.   the uterus is absent.
   d.   pregnancy has occurred.

14. (d,863)

14. Which of the following is a true statement:

   a.   Secondary amenorrhea is defined as a pathologic state.
   b.   Primary amenorrhea does not prevent the development of secondary sex characteristics.
   c.   Primary amenorrhea may be caused by pregnancy.
   d.   Turner syndrome is never seen with secondary amenorrhea.

15. (d,863)

15. _____ is a genetic disorder associated with primary amenorrhea.

   a.   Superfemale syndrome
   b.   Testicular feminizing syndrome
   c.   Gonadal dysgenesis
   d.   All of the above
   e.   None of the above

16. (b,864)

16. Clinical manifestations of a female patient include the following: irregular and/or heavy bleeding, passage of large clots, and anemia. This patient is experiencing:

   a.   premenstrual syndrome.
   b.   dysfunctional uterine bleeding.
   c.   polycystic ovarian syndrome.
   d.   primary dysmenorrhea.

17. (b,863)

17. By definition, dysfunctional uterine bleeding is abnormal uterine bleeding resulting from:

   a.   tumors.
   b.   changes in the menstrual cycle.
   c.   infections.
   d.   congenital abnormalities in uterine structure.

18. (d,864)

18. All of the following are true of women with polycystic ovarian syndrome *except*:

   a.   the hypothalamic-pituitary-ovarian axis is intact.
   b.   the ovary is without inherent defects.
   c.   the ovary is affected by excessive production of androgens by peripheral tissues.
   d.   there is no genetic basis.

19. (d,874)

19. A cystocele is a(n):

    a. inflammation of an ovarian cyst.
    b. infection of an ovarian cyst.
    c. malignant tumor of the vagina.
    d. displacement of the bladder.

20. (b,866,869)

20. Infection and inflammation of the female genitalia can be caused by both naturally occurring and foreign microorganisms. Possible resulting conditions include all of the following *except*:

    a. pelvic inflammatory disease.
    b. cystocele.
    c. cervicitis.
    d. bartholinitis.

21. (d,870)

21. Which of the following pelvic relaxation disorders is caused by factors relating to childbirth?

    a. urethrocele
    b. rectocele
    c. cystocele
    d. all of the above
    e. none of the above

22. (c,870)

22. _____ is the descent of the bladder and the anterior vaginal wall into the vaginal wall.

    a. Rectocele
    b. Vagocele
    c. Cystocele
    d. Urethrocele

23. (b,870)

23. _____ is the descent of the cervix or the entire uterus into the vaginal canal.

    a. Cervical prolapse
    b. Uterine prolapse
    c. Cervicoutero prolapse
    d. All of the above

24. (a,872)

24. A _____ develops from a dominant ovarian follicle that does not release its ovum but remains active or develops from a degenerating follicle whose fluid is not reabsorbed.

    a. follicular cyst
    b. corpus luteal cyst
    c. corpus albicans cyst
    d. atretic follicular cyst

25. (c,873)

25. _____ are benign uterine tumors that develop from smooth muscle cells in the myometrium and are commonly called uterine fibroids.

    a. Endometrial polyps
    b. Myometrial polyps
    c. Leiomyomas
    d. Adenomas

26. (a,874)

26. All of the following are clinical manifestations of endometriosis *except*:

    a. amenorrhea.
    b. infertility.
    c. dyspareunia.
    d. constipation.

27. (e,876)

27. Sites of implantation of endometrial tissue that respond to hormonal changes may be found in:

    a. cervix.
    b. lungs.
    c. extremities.
    d. pleural cavities.
    e. all of the above.

28. (e,874)

28. Medical therapies for endometriosis include suppressing ovulation with:

    a. GnRH agonist.
    b. laparoscopic removal.
    c. danazol.
    d. a and c
    e. a, b, and c

29. (c,876)

29. Which of the following represents the most commonly occurring cancer of the female reproductive tract?

    a. cervical cancer
    b. ovarian cancer
    c. endometrial cancer
    d. fallopian cancer

30. (e,877)

30. _____ is a risk factor for ovarian cancer.

    a. Having one or more first-degree relatives affected by ovarian cancer
    b. Having a personal history of breast cancer
    c. Having a high fat diet
    d. Having never been pregnant
    e. All of the above

31. (a,878)

31. In stage _____ ovarian cancer is limited to both ovaries.

    a. I
    b. II
    c. III
    d. IV

32. (a,880)

32. Urethritis is a common disorder of the male urethra. GU, a form of urethritis, is caused by:

    a. *Neisseria gonorrhea.*
    b. *Chlamydia trachomatis.*
    c. *Ureaplasma urealyticum.*
    d. b and c
    e. a, b, and c

33. (b,881)   33. _____ is a condition in which the foreskin cannot be retracted over the glans penis.

   a. Paraphimosis
   b. Phimosis
   c. Pre-phimosis
   d. Priapism

34. (d,881)   34. _____ is the "bent nail condition," a fibrotic condition that causes lateral curvature of the penis during erection.

   a. Phimosis
   b. Lateral phimosis
   c. Lateral paraphimosis
   d. Peyronie disease

35. (b,881)   35. _____ is inflammation of the glans penis.

   a. Glanitis
   b. Balanitis
   c. Priapism
   d. Hydroceleitis

36. (d,884)   36. Cryptorchidism can be defined as:

   a. a normal, developmental state of the testes.
   b. an abnormal state, in which there is overdevelopment of the testes.
   c. lack of a scrotum.
   d. problems with testicular descent.

37. (c, 885)   37. The risk of testicular cancer is 35 to 50 times greater for men with a history of:

   a. priapism.
   b. phymosis.
   c. cryptorchidism.
   d. testicular tortion.

38. (c,886)   38. _____ is the most common infectious cause of orchitis and usually affects postpubertal males.

   a. Herpes
   b. *E. coli*
   c. Mumps
   d. Cytomegalovirus

39. (e,886)   39. Testicular cancer, one of the leading fatal cancers in men in their twenties and thirties, can present with which of the following clinical manifestations?

   a. testicular enlargement
   b. hydrocele
   c. dull ache in the lower abdomen
   d. a and c
   e. a, b, and c

40. (d,891)   40. Prostate cancer:

   a. is more common in white males.
   b. usually occurs before age 50.
   c. is the leading cause of cancer in men.
   d. often causes no symptoms until it is far advanced.

41. (e,893)

41. Which of the following medications can lead to male sexual dysfunction?

    a.   hormones
    b.   antihypertensives
    c.   antidepressants
    d.   a and b
    e.   a, b, and c

42. (b,894)

42. Which of the following statements concerning galactorrhea is not correct?

    a.   It can occur in men.
    b.   It always involves both breasts.
    c.   It is generally the result of a pathophysiologic state originating somewhere in the body; however, not at the breasts.
    d.   Elevated prolactin levels, outside of pregnancy and childbirth, are the most common cause.

43. (d,903)

43. Which of the following is usually the first clinical manifestation of breast cancer?

    a.   dimpling
    b.   nipple discharge
    c.   chest pain
    d.   a painless lump

44. (a,907-908)

44. Parasitic STIs include all of the following *except*:

    a.   chlamydia.
    b.   pediculosis pubis.
    c.   scabies.
    d.   trichomoniasis.

45. (d,908)

45. Genital herpes may be caused by:

    a.   CMV.
    b.   HSV-1.
    c.   HSV-2.
    d.   b and c
    e.   a, b, and c

46. (c,908)

46. Condylomata acuminata, or genital warts, are caused by:

    a.   chlamydomonis.
    b.   adenovirus.
    c.   human papilloma virus.
    d.   HSV-1.

47. (a,908)

47. Treatments of HPV infection include:

    a.   topical application of 5-fluorouracil.
    b.   topical application of acyclovir.
    c.   systemic penicillin.
    d.   systemic tetracycline.
    e.   all of the above.

Olive Cole visits the clinic with a complaint of vaginal discharge and itching of the vulva, which became worse following her menstrual period. A vaginal examination reveals swelling and erythema of the vaginal wall and a copious gray-green discharge. A diagnosis of trichomoniasis is made.

48. (b,906)   48. The organism which causes trichomoniasis is:

    a.   a virus.
    b.   a protozoa.
    c.   a bacterium.
    d.   a spirochete.

49. (b,906)   49. Hepatitis _____ virus is known to be sexually transmitted.

    a.   A
    b.   B
    c.   non-A, non-B
    d.   none of the above

Matching

50. (c,879)   50. ____   sexual anorexia   a. painful, prolonged penile erection

51. (b,879)   51. ____   vaginismus   b. involuntary muscle spasm

52. (e,879)   52. ____   anorgasmia   c. decreased libido

53. (f,879)   53. ____   dyspareunia   d. retracted foreskin

54. (d,879)   54. ____   paraphimosis   e. orgasmic dysfunction

55. (a,879)   55. ____   priapism   f. painful intercourse

Short Answer

56. List four diseases that can affect sexual function.

57. What is a varicocele?

58. Why is testicular torsion a surgical emergency?

59. What is the most curable cancer of the male reproductive system?

60. What percentage of women will develop breast cancer during their lifetime?

Short Answers

56. Cerebral palsy, CVA diabetes, chronic renal failure, rheumatoid arthritis, SLE, MI, MS, spinal cord injury (880)
57. An abnormal dilation of a vein within the spermatic cord (883)
58. The testes will die in six hours if the blood supply is not reestablished. (885)
59. Testicular cancer—higher than 95% cure rate (886)
60. About 12.5% (900)

CHAPTER

33

Structure and Function of the Digestive System

Name _____

True/False

1. (T,926)   1. T   F   The two movements involved in intestinal motility are haustral segmentation and peristalsis.

2. (T,930)   2. T   F   Intestinal bacteria play a role in the formation of bile salts.

3. (F,918)   3. T   F   The salivary glands are under the direct control of the parasympathetic nervous system exclusively.

4. (F,921)   4. T   F   Vagal stimulation causes contraction of the stomach.

5. (F,922)   5. T   F   Normally there is regurgitation from the duodenum into the antrum.

6. (T,923)   6. T   F   The chief cells of the gastric glands secrete pepsinogen.

7. (T,922)   7. T   F   Gastric secretion is inhibited by unpleasant odors.

8. (F,926)   8. T   F   Insulin is required for active absorption of carbohydrates by the small intestine.

9. (F,938)   9. T   F   Aging generally causes an increase in both gastric motility and hydrochloric acid concentration.

Multiple Choice

10. (c,918)   10. The gastrointestinal tract provides all of the following processes *except*:

     a. absorption of digested food.
     b. chemical breakdown of food particles.
     c. micturition.
     d. mechanical breakdown of food particles.

11. (b,918)   11. Salivary alpha-amylase initiates the digestion of:

     a. proteins.
     b. carbohydrates.
     c. fats.
     d. amino acids.

12. (d,920)   12. Saliva contains_____,which helps prevent infection.

    a. IgG
    b. IgD
    c. IgE
    d. IgA

13. (a,918)   13. Ptyalin is an enzyme that initiates digestion of _____ in the mouth and stomach.

    a. carbohydrates
    b. proteins
    c. lipids
    d. a and b

14. (d,918)   14. The _____ nervous system controls the salivary glands.

    a. parasympathetic
    b. sympathetic
    c. somatic
    d. a and b
    e. a, b, and c

15. (b,918)   15. Atropine, a drug that inhibits the parasympathetic system, will cause the salivary glands to become:

    a. hyperactive.
    b. hypoactive.
    c. atrophied.
    d. enlarged.

16. (a,920)   16. Vagal innervation of the esophagus is least evident in the _____ third of the esophagus.

    a. upper
    b. middle
    c. lower
    d. none of the above

17. (d,920)   17. _____ increases muscle tone in the lower esophageal sphincter.

    a. Sympathetic stimulation
    b. Parasympathetic stimulation
    c. Vagal stimulation
    d. c and d
    e. a, b, and c

18. (c,920)   18. The _____ sphincter keeps air from entering the esophagus.

    a. cardiac
    b. lower esophageal
    c. upper esophageal
    d. a and b
    e. none of the above

19. (a,920)

19. Food moves down the esophagus via:

    a. peristalsis.
    b. haustral segmentation.
    c. retropulsion.
    d. defecation.

20. (c,921-922)

20. Autonomic and hormonal control are involved in:

    a. gastrointestinal motility and defecation.
    b. gastrointestinal motility and deglutition.
    c. gastrointestinal motility only.
    d. gastrointestinal motility and mastication.

21. (c,921)

21. The stomach is innervated by the _____ nervous system.

    a. sympathetic
    b. parasympathetic
    c. a and b

22. (e,921)

22. Stimulation of the stomach via _____ inhibits the muscle action of the stomach.

    a. secretin
    b. sympathetic nervous system
    c. parasympathetic nervous system
    d. gastrin
    e. a and b

23. (e,921)

23. Relaxation of the stomach is caused by:

    a. vagal fibers.
    b. gastrin.
    c. cholecystokinin.
    d. b and c.
    e. a, b, and c.

24. (b,922)

24. The _____ cells of the gastric glands secrete hydrochloric acid.

    a. chief
    b. parietal
    c. zymogenic
    d. none of the above

25. (d,923)

25. _____ stimulates the chief cells of the gastric glands to secrete pepsinogen during eating.

    a. Acetylcholine
    b. Gastrin
    c. Secretin
    d. All of the above

26. (c,922)

26. All of the following are functions of hydrochloric acid in the stomach *except*:

    a. dissolving food fibers.
    b. killing microorganisms.
    c. providing vitamin B_{12} absorption.
    d. activating pepsin.

27. (a,924)

27. Which of the following phases of acid secretion by the stomach involves stimulation by antici-pation and swallowing?

    a. cephalic phase
    b. gastric phase
    c. intestinal phase
    d. a and b
    e. a, b, and c

28. (a,924)

28. Just thinking about food can stimulate gastric secretion; secretions stimulated in this way are considered part of the _____ phase of gastric secretion

    a. cephalic
    b. caudal
    c. gastric
    d. intestinal

29. (e,924)

29. _____ is a powerful stimulus for gastric secretion.

    a. The presence of food in the stomach
    b. Stretching of the stomach
    c. Smelling food
    d. Thinking about food
    e. all of the above

30. (b,924)

30. The ileum and jejunum are suspended by folds of the peritoneum, the _____, that contain an extensive vascular and nervous network.

    a. myenteric plexus
    b. mesentery
    c. Auerbach's folds
    d. Meissner plexus

31. (d,929)

31. Sugars are absorbed in:

    a. the duodenum.
    b. the jejunum.
    c. the ileum.
    d. a and b.
    e. a, b, and c.

32. (a,926)

32. Digested fats leave the intestine, initially via the:

    a. lacteals.
    b. villi.
    c. hepatic portal veins.
    d. celiac veins.

33. (d,927)

33. Which of the following statements is false?

    a. Maltase from the small intestine helps to break down maltose.
    b. Trypsin is involved in protein digestion.
    c. Pepsin activation requires hydrochloric acid.
    d. Pancreatic amylases break down oligosaccharides.

34. (d,927)

34. _____ carries out hydrolysis of proteins in the small intestine.

a. Trypsin
b. Chymotrypsin
c. Brush border enzymes
d. all of the above

35. (d,929)

35. Which of the following is not a step in the absorption of fats?

a. emulsification
b. lipolysis
c. micelle formation
d. amino acid hydrolysis

36. (d,928)

36. All of the following water-soluble vitamins require sodium-dependent active transport for absorption *except*:

a. vitamin B_6.
b. vitamin B_1.
c. vitamin C.
d. vitamin B_{12}.

37. (a,926)

37. Distension of the ileum with chyme causes:

a. the ileogastric reflex.
b. the intestino-intestinal reflex.
c. the gastroileal reflex.
d. the intestinal reflex.

38. (a,926)

38. The _____ inhibits gastric motility when the ileum becomes over-distended.

a. intestino-intestinal reflex
b. ileogastric reflex
c. intestinal reflex
d. gastroileal reflex

39. (c,928)

39. The _____ sphincter controls the movement of chyme from the sigmoid colon into the rectum.

a. Odi
b. ileocecal
c. O'Beirne
d. internal anal

40. (a,929)

40. The _____ reflex initiates propulsion in the entire colon, usually during or immediately after eating.

a. gastrocolic
b. ileocolic
c. duodenalcolic
d. cephalocolic

41. (e,933-935)

41. Functions of the liver include:

a. digestive
b. immunologic
c. vascular
d. a and c
e. a, b, and c

42. The sinusoids of the liver are lined in part by _____ cells, which are phagocytic.

    a.   Alice
    b.   Kupffer
    c.   Ishmael
    d.   Moses

43. The primary bile acids are synthesized from _____ by hepatocytes lining the bile canaliculi.

    a.   lecithin
    b.   fatty acids
    c.   cholesterol
    d.   testosterone

44. In the liver unconjugated bilirubin moves from the plasma in the sinusoids into the hepatocytes where it is converted into water-soluble:

    a.   bilirubin.
    b.   biliverdin.
    c.   conjugated bilirubin.
    d.   urobilinogen.

45. The function of the acinar cells of the pancreas is:

    a.   to secrete bicarbonate.
    b.   to secrete enzymes.
    c.   to secrete water.
    d.   to secrete electrolytes.

46. During the cephalic and gastric phases of digestion, gallbladder contraction is mediated by cholinergic branches of the:

    a.   sympathetic nervous system.
    b.   somatic nervous system.
    c.   vagus nerves.
    d.   glossopharyngeal nerves.

47. The exocrine portion of the pancreas contains:

    a.   beta cells.
    b.   alpha cells.
    c.   ducts.
    d.   islets of Langerhans.

Matching

48. (f,922)

49. (c,922)

50. (b,922)

51. (a,922)

52. (d,923)

53. (e,922)

48. ___ gastrin

49. ___ motilin

50. ___ secretin

51. ___ cholecystokinin

52. ___ pepsin

53. ___ ptyalin

a. stimulates gallbladder to eject bile

b. stimulates pancreas to secrete bicarbonate

c. increases gastrointestinal motility

d. digests proteins

e. initiates carbohydrate digestion

f. stimulates gastric glands to secrete hydrochloric acid and pepsinogen

Short Answer

54. List the components of saliva.

55. List the three functional areas of the stomach and give their locations.

56. Define retropulsion.

57. List two aerobic and two anaerobic bacteria in the gut.

58. What are the three accessory organs of digestion?

59. How much bile is secreted per day?

60. List three laboratory tests that measure pancreatic function.

Short Answers

54. Water, mucus, sodium, bicarbonate, chloride, potassium, IgA (918)
55. Fundus—upper portion; body—middle portion; antrum—lower portion (921)
56. As food approaches the pylorus, the velocity of peristaltic waves increases. This forces the contents back toward the body of the stomach. This process effectively mixes food with digestive juices, and the oscillation causes large food particles to be broken down. (922)
57. Aerobes: streptococci, lactobacilli, staphylococci, enterobacteria
    Anaerobes: bacteroides, clostridia, anaerobic lactobacilli, coliforms (930)
58. Liver, gallbladder, exocrine pancreas (930)
59. 700 to 1200 ml/day (930)
60. Serum amylase, serum lipase, urine amylase, secretin test, stool fat (938)

Alterations of Digestive Function

Name _____

True/False

1. (T,943)   1. T   F   Anorexia is the lack of desire to eat despite physiologic stimuli that would normally produce hunger.

2. (T,943)   2. T   F   Because patterns of bowel evacuation differ greatly among individuals, constipation must be individually defined.

3. (T,944)   3. T   F   Abdominal pain can be parietal, visceral, or referred.

4. (F,948)   4. T   F   Hiatal hernia occurs when the intestine protrudes into the umbilicus.

5. (F,950)   5. T   F   Chronic gastritis of the fundus occurs more frequently than antral gastritis.

6. (F,952)   6. T   F   The incidence of duodenal ulcers is approximately the same among men and women.

7. (F,954)   7. T   F   Exacerbations of duodenal ulcers tend to occur in the summer and winter.

8. (F,963)   8. T   F   Jaundice is the most common cause of ascites.

Multiple Choice

9. (e,943)   9. All of the following stimulate the vomiting reflex *except*:

   a.   severe pain.
   b.   distention of the stomach.
   c.   copper salts in the duodenum.
   d.   trauma to the ovaries.
   e.   diarrhea.

10. (c,943)   10. _____ vomiting is caused by direct stimulation of the vomiting center by direct neurological lesions involving the brain stem.

   a.   Retch
   b.   Periodic
   c.   Projectile
   d.   Duodenal

11. (c,943)

11. Normal bowel habits range from two or three evacuations per day to one per:

    a.   day.
    b.   two days.
    c.   week.
    d.   month.

12. (b,943)

12. Opiate drugs _____ constipation.

    a.   relieve
    b.   exacerbate
    c.   most likely have no effect on

13. (a,943)

13. Which of the following is not a cause of constipation?

    a.   hyperthyroidism
    b.   certain drugs
    c.   sedentary life style
    d.   low-residue diet

14. (c,944)

14. The adult intestine processes approximately _____ liter(s) of luminal content per day, of which 99% of the fluid is normally reabsorbed.

    a.   1
    b.   6
    c.   9
    d.   12

15. (b,944)

15. Bill has been diagnosed with diabetic neuropathy. Which of the following would be expected due to this condition?

    a.   osmotic diarrhea
    b.   secretory diarrhea
    c.   motility diarrhea
    d.   a and c
    e.   a, b, and c

16. (b,944)

16. If a person lacks the enzyme lactase and ingests lactose, the lactose will not be hydrolyzed and absorbed into the intestinal wall; the type of diarrhea that results is _____ diarrhea.

    a.   motility
    b.   osmotic
    c.   secretory
    d.   a and b
    e.   a, b, and c

17. (a,944)

17. _____ pain arises from a stimulus acting on an abdominal organ. It is usually felt near the midline in the epigastrium, midabdomen, or lower abdomen.

    a.   Visceral
    b.   Abdominal
    c.   Parietal
    d.   Retroperitoneal

18. (c,945)   18. Frank bleeding of the rectum is called:

    a. melena.
    b. occult bleeding.
    c. hematochezia.
    d. hematemesis.

19. (c,945)   19. Functional dysphagia is caused by:

    a. intrinsic mechanical obstruction.
    b. extrinsic mechanical obstruction.
    c. neural or muscular disorder.
    d. a and b.
    e. a, b, and c.

20. (a,945)   20. Achalasia results from:

    a. neural dysfunction.
    b. intrinsic mechanical obstruction.
    c. extrinsic mechanical obstruction.
    d. none of the above.

21. (b,947)   21. Reflux esophagitis may be defined as:

    a. an immune response to gastroesophageal reflux.
    b. an inflammatory response to gastroesophageal reflux.
    c. a congenital anomaly.
    d. a secretory response to gastroesophageal reflux.

22. (c,948)   22. _____ is the narrowing of the opening between the stomach and the duodenum.

    a. Ileocecal obstruction
    b. Hiatal hernia
    c. Pyloric obstruction
    d. Hiatal obstruction

23. (e,949-950) 23. Intestinal obstruction may be caused by:

    a. mechanical obstruction of the lumen.
    b. inflammatory disorders.
    c. adhesions.
    d. a and b.
    e. a, b, and c.

24. (a,950)   24. Which of the following is associated with chronic fundal gastritis?

    a. pernicious anemia
    b. osmotic diarrhea
    c. increased acid secretion
    d. decreased gastrin secretion
    e. a, b, and c

25. (e,952)

25. Peptic ulcers are located in the mucosa of the:

   a.   stomach.
   b.   esophagus.
   c.   duodenum.
   d.   a and b.
   e.   a, b, and c.

26. (d,952)

26. _____ is the primary cause of duodenal ulcers.

   a.   Hypersecretion of acid by the stomach
   b.   Hypersecretion of pepsin by the stomach
   c.   Hypersecretion of acid by the duodenum
   d.   *H. pylori* infection

27. (c,952)

27. A peptic ulcer may occur in all of the following areas *except*:

   a.   stomach.
   b.   upper small intestine.
   c.   jejunum.
   d.   lower esophagus.

28. (b,955)

28. _____ ulcer is a stress ulcer that is associated with severe head trauma or brain surgery.

   a.   Addison
   b.   Cushing
   c.   Ischemic
   d.   Curling

29. (a,958)

29. A patient is complaining of abdominal pain, diarrhea, and bloody stools. A possible diagnosis would be:

   a.   ulcerative colitis.
   b.   hiatal hernia.
   c.   pyloric obstruction.
   d.   achalasia.

30. (e,957)

30. Clinical manifestations of bile salt deficiencies are related to poor absorption of:

   a.   fat-soluble vitamins.
   b.   water-soluble vitamins.
   c.   fats.
   d.   a and b.
   e.   a and c.

31. (c,960)

31. Which of the following is not a true statement concerning appendicitis?

   a.   It is the most common surgical emergency.
   b.   Epigastric or periumbilical pain is often present.
   c.   Obstruction of the lumen causes a decrease in intraluminal pressure which may produce appendicitis.
   d.   The inflammation may progress to gangrene.

32. (b,975)

32. The second most common type of cancer in the U.S. is:

    a.   liver cancer.
    b.   colorectal cancer.
    c.   lung cancer.
    d.   gastric cancer.
    e.   pancreatic cancer.

33. (d,963)

33. Which of the following is not a cause for hepatic portal hypertension?

    a.   thrombosis
    b.   hepatitis
    c.   cardiac disorders
    d.   disorders of the spleen

34. (e,963)

34. Long-term portal hypertension may result in:

    a.   hepatic encephalopathy.
    b.   splenomegaly.
    c.   ascites.
    d.   varices.
    e.   all of the above

35. (c,963)

35. The most common clinical manifestation of portal hypertension is:

    a.   rectal bleeding.
    b.   duodenal bleeding.
    c.   esophageal bleeding.
    d.   intestinal bleeding.

36. (b,966)

36. Which of the following types of jaundice is due to an increase in the rate of red blood cell breakdown?

    a.   obstructive jaundice
    b.   hemolytic jaundice
    c.   hepatocellular jaundice
    d.   a and b
    e.   a, b, and c

37. (b,967)

37. Hepatitis A is characterized by:

    a.   an incubation period of 60-180 days.
    b.   an acute onset.
    c.   a positive carrier state.
    d.   a sexual mode of transmission.

38. (d,970)

38. Hepatic fat accumulation is seen in:

    a.   biliary cirrhosis.
    b.   metabolic cirrhosis.
    c.   postnecrotic cirrhosis.
    d.   alcohol cirrhosis.

39. (d,975-976) 39. Clinical manifestations of colorectal cancer include all of the following *except*:

a. bloody stools.
b. pain.
c. anemia.
d. jaundice.

Matching

40. (d,967)   40. ___ hepatitis A   a. chronic active form predisposes to cirrhosis

41. (a,968)   41. ___ hepatitis B   b. may be associated with fulminant hepititis

42. (e,967)   42. ___ hepatitis C   c. fecal-oral transmission; can be chronic

43. (c,967)   43. ___ hepatitis D   d. acute onset with fever

44. (f,967)   44. ___ hepatitis E   e. severity unknown

45. (b,967)   45. ___ hepatitis G   f. severe in pregnant women

Short Answer

46. List the two major causes of duodenal ulcers.

47. Which inflammatory bowel disease tends to run in families?

48. List four theories of obesity.

49. List the long-term effects of portal hypertension.

50. What is the most common cause of chronic pancreatitis.

51. What are the three phases of hepatitis?

52. People with type A blood are at increased risk for what gastrointestinal cancer?

53. Familial adenomatous polyposis is a risk factor for which gastrointestinal cancer?

54. Mortality from pancreatic cancer is nearly _____ %.

55. List the four characteristics of anorexia nervosa.

Short Answers

46. *H. pylori* infection and use of nonsteroidal antiinflammatory drugs (952)
47. Crohn disease (959)
48. Genetic theory, fat-cell theory, lipoprotein-lipase theory, lipostatic theory, thermogenic theory, sodium-potassium-ATP-ASE pump theory, diabetes-associated theory, psychologic causation theory (961)
49. Varices, splenomegaly, ascites, hepatic encephalopathy (963)
50. Chronic alcohol abuse (972)
51. Prodromal phase, icteric phase, recovery phase (968)
52. Cancer of the stomach (974)
53. Colorectal cancer (975)
54. 100% (979)
55. Fear of becoming obese despite progressive weight loss; distorted body image; body weight 15% below normal because of refusal to eat; absence of three consecutive menstrual periods. (961)

Alterations of Digestive Function in Children

Name _____

True/False

1. (T,988)

1. T F In most cases, cleft lip and cleft palate are caused by multiple factors, both genetic and environmental.

2. (T,989)

2. T F Esophageal atresia in the newborn is treated by surgical procedures.

3. (F,990)

3. T F Pyloric stenosis is more common in female children than in male.

4. (F,991)

4. T F Meconium is an abnormal formation of fluid in the intestine of the newborn.

5. (F,992)

5. T F Congenital aganglionic megacolon is caused by a malformation of the sympathetic nervous system. It is the absence of the intramural ganglion cells in the enteric nerve plexuses.

6. (T,997)

6. T F Failure to thrive is a nutritional disorder having both organic and nonorganic causes.

7. (F,1000)

7. T F Biliary atresia always shows a definite genetic cause.

8. (F,1000)

8. T F Children with hepatitis A demonstrate prolonged periods of jaundice.

9. (F,1001)

9. T F Most forms of chronic liver disease in children can progress to cirrhosis and often do so.

10. (T,1001)

10. T F People with galactosemia have hepatic clinical manifestations.

11. (T,1001)

11. T F Wilson disease is an autosomal recessive disease affecting copper metabolism in children and young adults.

Multiple Choice

12. (d,988)

12. Severe forms of incomplete fusion of the nasomedial or intermaxillary process during embryonic development causes:

    a. cleft palate.
    b. sinus dysfunction.
    c. cleft lip.
    d. a and c.
    e. a, b, and c.

13. (d,988-989)   13. Children with cleft palate tend to suffer from:

    a.   repeated infections of the paranasal sinuses.
    b.   excessive dental decay.
    c.   cleft lip.
    d.   all of the above.

14. (a,990)   14. Increased gastrin secretion by the mother in the last trimester of pregnancy may cause:

    a.   pyloric stenosis.
    b.   meconium ileus.
    c.   esophageal atresia.
    d.   galactosemia.

15. (c,989)   15. In at least _____ % of infants with esophageal defects, other congenital anomalies are present as well.

    a.   10
    b.   20
    c.   30
    d.   90

16. (b,990)   16. _____ is (are) routinely used to detect the hypertrophied pyloric muscles and the narrowed pyloric canal, characteristic of pyloric stenosis.

    a.   Contrast x-ray examinations
    b.   Sonography
    c.   MRI
    d.   Encephalogram

17. (a,990)   17. In _____ the developing colon remains in the upper right quadrant instead of moving to its normal location.

    a.   malrotation
    b.   ileocecal displacement
    c.   duodenal obstruction
    d.   none of the above

18. (b,991)   18. _____ is an intestinal obstruction caused by meconium formed in utero that is abnormally sticky and adheres firmly to the mucosa of the small intestine.

    a.   Meconium cecum
    b.   Meconium ileus
    c.   Meconium duodenum
    d.   Meconium vivax

19. (c,991)   19. Meconium ileus is often associated with:

    a.   muscular dystrophy.
    b.   cerebral palsy.
    c.   cystic fibrosis.
    d.   multiple sclerosis.

20. (b,991)

20. _____ is a functional obstruction of the colon caused by inadequate motility.

    a. Congenital ganglionic microcolon
    b. Congenital aganglionic megacolon
    c. Congenital hyperganglionic megacolon
    d. Congenital hyperparasympathetic megacolon

21. (b,992)

21. Hirschsprung disease involves a neural malformation in which of the following?

    a. the central nervous system
    b. the parasympathetic nervous system
    c. the sympathetic nervous system
    d. the somatic nervous system

22. (d,992)

22. Intussusception may be defined as:

    a. gastric folding.
    b. esophageal spasms.
    c. rectal obstruction in the newborn.
    d. intestinal invagination.

23. (c,992)

23. An intestinal obstruction called _____ occurs when the ileum collapses through the ileocecal valve and is invaginated into the cecum and part of the ascending colon.

    a. prolapse
    b. introlapse
    c. intussusception
    d. imperforation

24. (b,994)

24. The pathophysiologic triad that is the hallmark of cystic fibrosis includes all of the following *except*:

    a. increased respiratory mucus production.
    b. excessive salivation.
    c. pancreatic enzyme deficiency.
    d. elevated sodium and chloride concentrations in sweat.

25. (d,994)

25. Fibrocystic disease of the pancreas, also called _____, is a genetically transmitted disease that involves many organs and systems and usually causes death in childhood or young adulthood.

    a. cystic fibrosis
    b. mucoviscidosis
    c. muscular dystrophy
    d. a and b
    e. b and c

26. (b,994)

26. Hallmarks of cystic fibrosis include all of the following *except*:

    a. pancreatic enzyme deficiency.
    b. underproduction of mucus in the respiratory tract.
    c. abnormally elevated sodium and chloride concentrations in the sweat.
    d. maldigestion.

27. (b,996)

27. An infant is demonstrating diarrhea, vomiting, and abdominal pain. A possible diagnosis would be:

    a.   necrotizing enterocolitis.
    b.   gluten-sensitive enteropathy.
    c.   gastroesophageal reflux.
    d.   meconium ileus.

28. (e,999)

28. Prolonged diarrhea is more severe in children than adults because:

    a.   dehydration can occur more rapidly in children.
    b.   fluid reserves are smaller in children.
    c.   children have a lower fluid volume intake.
    d.   a and c.
    e.   a, b, and c.

29. (b,999)

29. Increased bilirubin production, impaired hepatic uptake and excretion of bilirubin, and reabsorption of bilirubin in the small intestine can each lead to:

    a.   biliary hypertrophy.
    b.   physiologic jaundice of the newborn.
    c.   hepatitis A.
    d.   infantile cirrhosis.

30. (d,1000)

30. _____ is a congenital malformation characterized by the absence or obstruction of intra-hepatic or extrahepatic bile ducts.

    a.   Hepatic atresia
    b.   Portal atresia
    c.   Sinusoidal atresia
    d.   Biliary atresia

31. (e,1000)

31. Progressive obstruction of the flow of bile may lead to:

    a.   progressive jaundice.
    b.   clay-colored stools.
    c.   liver failure.
    d.   a and c.
    e.   a, b, and c.

32. (b,1000)

32. The primary clinical manifestation of biliary atresia is:

    a.   kernicterus.
    b.   jaundice.
    c.   hypobilirubinemia.
    d.   all of the above

33. (d,1000)

33. Hepatitis _____ in children is primarily associated with blood transfusions.

    a.   A
    b.   B
    c.   C
    d.   a and c
    e.   a, b, and c

34. (d,1001)

34. _____ is a basic cause of portal hypertension in children.

   a. Increased resistance to blood flow within the portal system
   b. Increased volume of portal blood flow
   c. Cardiac disease
   d. a and b
   e. a, b, and c

35. (c,1002)

35. Clinical manifestations of portal hypertension in children include all of the following *except*:

   a. splenomegaly.
   b. ascites.
   c. jaundice.
   d. upper gastrointestinal bleeding.

36. (c,1002)

36. _____ is a clinical sign of portal hypertension.

   a. Right heart failure
   b. Pulmonary edema
   c. Splenomegaly
   d. Diarrhea

37. (a,1001)

37. Galactosemia is characterized as an:

   a. autosomal recessive trait.
   b. autosomal dominant trait.
   c. X-linked recessive trait.
   d. X-linked dominant trait.

38. (e,1002)

38. Early identification and treatment for metabolic disorders is important because:

   a. permanent damage to vital organs can be prevented.
   b. genetic counseling can begin.
   c. complications can be minimized.
   d. a and c.
   e. a, b, and c.

39. (c,989)

39. Polyhydramnios is seen in 14%–90% of mothers whose newborns have:

   a. cleft lip and palate.
   b. pyloric stenosis.
   c. esophageal malformation.
   d. malrotation.

40. (c,992)

40. Anorectal malformations that cause complete destruction are known as:
   a. intussusception.
   b. imperforate anus.
   c. anal stenosis.
   d. megacolon.

Matching

41. (c, 1001)   41. ___   defect in copper excretion   a. galactosemia

42. (a, 1001)   42. ___   cannot make gluscose   b. fructosemia

43. (b, 1001)   43. ___   occurs when breast milk is replaced   c. Wilson disease
                                with cow's milk

Short Answer

44. What chromosomal defect is associated with cleft lip and palate?

45. When do symptoms of pyloric stenosis begin?

46. Meconiim ileus is often associated with _____.

47. What is the usual manifestation of Hirschsprung disease?

48. Currant jelly stools are seen in _____.

49. _____ has been associated with sudden infant death syndrome.

50. What are the two most common types of malnutrition in children?

Short Answers

44. Trisomy 13 (988)
45. 2 to 3 weeks after birth (990)
46. Cystic fibrosis (991)
47. Mild to severe constipation (992)
48. Intussusception (993)
49. Gastroesophageal reflux (994)
50. Kwashiorkor and marasmus (997)

CHAPTER

36

Structure and Function of the Musculoskeletal System

Name _____

True/False

1. (F,1010)	1. T F The human skeleton contains 200 bones.
2. (F,1007)	2. T F Bone cells enable bone to grow and change shape up until the time of puberty only.
3. (F,1010)	3. T F Nerves may be found in the periosteum but not within the bone itself.
4. (F,1010)	4. T F Both compact and spongy bone are present in all bones.
5. (T,1012)	5. T F Osteoclasts are involved in the remodeling of bone.
6. (F,1016)	6. T F A procallus is involved in microscopic repair of bone.
7. (T,1016)	7. T F The most movable and most complex joints are synovial joints.

Multiple Choice

8. (c,1009)

8. The organic components of bones, the bone matrix, consist of _____ and other organic molecules.

   a. calcium
   b. phosphate
   c. collagen
   d. magnesium
   e. a and b

9. (b,1009)

9. _____ are osteoblasts that are found within mineralized bone matrix.

   a. Osteoclasts
   b. Osteocytes
   c. Fibrocytes

10. (b,1009)

10. Which of the following cells function to maintain bone matrix?

   a. osteoclasts
   b. osteocytes
   c. osteoblasts
   d. none of the above

11. (b,1009)

11. _____ are large cells that digest bone.

   a. Osteoblasts
   b. Osteoclasts
   c. Osteocytes
   d. Fibrocytes

12. (b,1009)

12. Which of the following is not part of the bone matrix?

   a. collagen fibers
   b. cellulose fibers
   c. proteoglycans
   d. glycoproteins

13. (c,1009)

13. _____ is a glycoprotein found in bone.

   a. Collagen
   b. Elastin
   c. Alphaglycoprotein
   d. Osteocalcin

14. (b,1009)

14. Which of the following glycoproteins binds to calcium in the bones?

   a. proteoglycans
   b. sialoprotein
   c. osteodentin
   d. albumin

15. (a,1009)

15. Osteocalcin is a:

   a. glycoprotein.
   b. hormone.
   c. mineral.
   d. vitamin.

16. (a,1010)

16. Bone is made up of two types of osseous tissue: compact (cortical bone) and spongy (cancellous bone). The major difference between the two types is:

   a. the organization of the structural elements.
   b. the location within the body.
   c. the activating chemicals in each.
   d. the deactivating chemicals in each.

17. (d,1010)

17. Compact bone is highly organized, solid, and extremely strong. The basic structural unit in compact bone is:

   a. small channels called canaliculae.
   b. osteocytes within the lacunae.
   c. tiny spaces within the lacunae.
   d. central Haversian canal.

18. (b,1010)

18. Which of the following statements about spongy bone tissue is not true?

   a. It is less complex than compact bone tissue.
   b. The lamellae are arranged in concentric layers instead of a trabecular meshwork.
   c. Osteocyte-containing lacunae are interconnected by canaliculae.
   d. The presence of bone marrow allows nourishment of the osteocytes.

19. (e,1010)

19. _____ is (are) not present in spongy bone.

    a.   Haversian canal
    b.   Concentric layers of matrix
    c.   Canaliculi
    d.   a and c
    e.   None are present in spongy bone.

20. (a,1010)

20. The outer layer of the periosteum contains blood vessels and nerves, some of which penetrate to the inner structures of the bone via:

    a.   Volkmann's canals.
    b.   canaliculi.
    c.   Sharpey canals.
    d.   none of the above.

21. (d,1012)

21. The human skeleton consists of 206 bones which comprise the axial skeleton (80 bones) and the appendicular skeleton (126 bones). Each bone can be classified by shape. Which of the following shapes is not an accepted classification?

    a.   long
    b.   flat
    c.   short (cuboidal)
    d.   regular

22. (c,1012)

22. After puberty the epiphyseal plate calcifies and the epiphysis and _____ merge.

    a.   epiphyseal line
    b.   epiphyseal plate
    c.   metaphysis
    d.   articular cartilage

23. (d,1012)

23. A stimulus for a bone remodeling cycle may be a:

    a.   hormone.
    b.   physical stressor.
    c.   vitamin.
    d.   any of the above

24. (c,1012)

24. The internal structure of bone is maintained by remodeling, a three-phase process in which existing bone is resorbed and new bone is laid down to replace it. Remodeling is done by clusters of bone cells called:

    a.   precursor stimulating cells.
    b.   osteoclastic cutting cones.
    c.   basic multicellular units.
    d.   Haversian system cells.

25. (e,1013)

25. The remodeling process can repair microscopic bone injuries, but gross injuries, such as fractures and surgical wounds, heal by the same stages as soft tissue injuries, including:

    a.   hematoma formation.
    b.   procallus and callus formation.
    c.   bone replacement.
    d.   a and c.
    e.   a, b, and c.

26. (d,1014)

26. The site where two or more bones are attached is called a joint or articulation. Joints are classified on the degree of movement they permit the connecting tissue they hold together. Which of the following terms describes a freely movable joint?

    a. synarthrosis
    b. amphiarthrosis
    c. biarthrosis
    d. diarthrosis

27. (b,1014)

27. The elbow joint is an example of a(n):

    a. amphiarthrosis.
    b. diarthrosis.
    c. synarthrosis.
    d. all of the above

28. (c,1014, 1016)

28. A joint in which bone is united directly to bone by fibrous connective tissue is called a fibrous joint. A joint united by either fibrocartilage or hyaline cartilage is called a cartilaginous joint. Which of the following are subclassifications of a cartilaginous joint?

    a. sutures and gomphosis
    b. syndesmosis and gomphosis
    c. symphysis and synchondrosis
    d. gomphosis and synchondrosis

29. (a,1015)

29. Synovial joints are the most movable and complex joints in the body. Which of the following is not a synovial joint?

    a. a hinge type which connects two vertebrae
    b. a spheroid type found in the shoulder
    c. a hinge type found in the elbow
    d. a gliding type found in the hand

30. (c,1015)

30. The teeth in the maxilla or mandible are examples of a(n):

    a. amphiarthrosis.
    b. diarthrosis.
    c. synarthrosis.
    d. all of the above

31. (e,1016)

31. _____ joints are the most movable and most complex joints of the body.

    a. Synovial
    b. Synchondrosis
    c. Gomphosis
    d. Diarthrotic
    e. a and d

32. (d,1020)

32. The joint capsule is richly supplied with:

    a. blood vessels.
    b. nerves.
    c. lymphatic vessels.
    d. all of the above.

33. (b,1016) | 33. Which of the following statements about muscle is not true?

    a. muscle comprises 50% of an adult's body weight and 40% of a child's
    b. muscle is 75% water, 20% protein, and 5% organic and inorganic compounds
    c. 32% of all protein stores for energy and metabolism are contained in muscle
    d. none of the above
    e. a, b, and c

34. (d,1017) | 34. Skeletal muscle is controlled directly by the central nervous system via a system of motor and sensory nerve fibers. Which of the following terms is not used to describe skeletal muscle?

    a. voluntary
    b. striated
    c. extrafusal
    d. contractile

35. (b,1016) | 35. Costal cartilage is located between:

    a. the vertebra.
    b. the ribs and sternum.
    c. the sutures of the skull.
    d. the facial bones.

36. (a,1014) | 36. Generally, fibrous joints are:

    a. immovable.
    b. slightly movable.
    c. freely movable.
    d. moderately movable.

37. (b,1022) | 37. The type of muscle fiber in a motor unit determines whether the muscle nerve is fast or slow. Muscle fibers are termed type I (red) or type II (white). Which of the following characteristics is *not* applicable to a type I fiber?

    a. slow contraction speed
    b. low resistance to fatigue
    c. profuse capillary supply
    d. oxidative metabolism

38. (a,1022) | 38. Which of the following characteristics is not applicable to a type II fiber?

    a. slow contraction speed
    b. low resistance to fatigue
    c. rapid firing frequency
    d. glycolysis metabolism

39. (d,1022) | 39. The lowest ratio of motor units per unit of muscle would be seen in which of the following:

    a. muscles that move the lower leg
    b. back muscles
    c. upper arm muscles
    d. muscles that move the fingers

40. (c,1021)

40. Which of the following is the functional unit of a muscle contraction?

   a.   motor unit
   b.   basement membrane
   c.   myofibril
   d.   ribosome

41. (d,1023)

41. The myofibrils contain sarcomeres that consist mainly of _____ muscle proteins.

   a.   actin
   b.   myosin
   c.   collagen
   d.   a and b
   e.   a, b, and c

42. (d,1024)

42. Which of the following correctly describes a muscle contraction's four-step process?

   a.   coupling, contraction, relaxation, excitation
   b.   contraction, relaxation, excitation, coupling
   c.   relaxation, excitation, coupling, contraction
   d.   excitation, coupling, contraction, relaxation

43. (c,1025)

43. _____ ions directly control the contraction of muscles.

   a.   Sodium
   b.   Potassium
   c.   Calcium
   d.   Magnesium

44. (b,1026)

44. In _____ contractions of muscles, the muscle maintains a constant length as tension is increased.

   a.   isotonic
   b.   isometric
   c.   hypertonic
   d.   hypotonic

45. (b,1026)

45. Which of the following describes a functional muscle contraction in which the muscle contracts but the limb does not move?

   a.   isotonic contraction
   b.   isometric contraction
   c.   eccentric contraction
   d.   concentric contraction

Matching

46. (c,1020)

46. ___ fibrous connective tissue that covers the ends of bones

a. synovial membrane

b. synovial fluid

47. (a,1020)

47. ___ smooth, delicate inner lining of joint muscle

c. articular cartilage

48. (b,1020)

48. ___ superinflated plasma that lubricates joint surfaces

d. joint cavity

49. (d,1020)

49. ___ enclosed, fluid-filled space between two bones

Short Answer

50. The growth plate in bones is named the _____.

51. List the three types of joints based on movement.

52. List the three layers of fascia.

53. List four movements of the foot.

54. List three nonprotein constituents of muscle.

55. List two types of muscle movements.

Short Answers

50. Epiphysis (1012)
51. Synarthrosis, amphiarthrosis, diarthrosis (1014)
52. Epimysium, perimysium, endomysium (1017)
53. Dorsiflexion, plantar flexion, inversion, eversion (1018)
54. Nitrogen, creatine, phosphocreatine, purines, uric acid, amino acids (1024)
55. Isometric, isotonic (1026)

Alterations of Musculoskeletal Function

Name _____

True/False

1. (T,1032) 1. T F A fracture in which the bone breaks into two or more fragments is termed a comminuted fracture.

2. (T,1033) 2. T F Insufficiency fractures occur in bones lacking the normal ability to deform and recover.

3. (T,1040) 3. T F In osteoporosis the bone that remains is histologically and biochemically normal.

4. (T,1043) 4. T F In osteomalacia the remodeling cycle proceeds normally through osteoid formation, but mineral calcification and deposition does not occur.

5. (F,1045) 5. T F Paget disease can occur in any bone, but it most often affects the appendicular skeleton.

6. (T,1046) 6. T F Osteomyelitis is a bone infection caused by bacteria; however fungi, parasites, and viruses can also cause bone infection.

7. (T,1051) 7. T F Inflammatory joint disease (arthritis) can be infectious or noninfectious.

8. (F,1053) 8. T F The onset of rheumatoid arthritis is always insidious.

9. (T,1066) 9. T F Alcohol abuse is the most common cause of toxic myopathy.

Multiple Choice

10. (d,1032) 10. The incidence of fractures of the pelvis are highest in:

    a. preadolescent boys.
    b. adolescent boys.
    c. adolescent girls.
    d. elderly adults.

11. (b,1033)

11. Mrs. Angie Aguardo, a 65-year-old Hispanic woman, is admitted to the hospital with a pathologic, compound, oblique fracture of the femur. Which of the following is true?

    a.   The fracture line runs parallel to the bone.
    b.   The fracture line runs diagonally to the shaft of the bone.
    c.   The fracture line runs perpendicular to the bone.
    d.   The fracture line runs vertically to the shaft of the bone.

12. (d,1033)

12. All of the following are commonly associated with a pathologic fracture *except*:

    a.   tumors, infections, osteoporosis.
    b.   break at the site of a preexisting abnormality.
    c.   weakening of bone cortex.
    d.   higher than normal break threshold.

13. (c,1033)

13. _____ is a fracture at a site of a preexisting bone abnormality, usually by a force that would not normally cause a fracture.

    a.   Idiopathic fracture
    b.   Iatrogenic fracture
    c.   Pathologic fracture
    d.   None of the above

14. (c,1033)

14. _____ fractures usually occur in individuals who engage in a new activity that is both strenuous and repetitive.

    a.   Insufficiency
    b.   Greenstick
    c.   Fatigue
    d.   Compound

15. (a,1034)

15. Transchondral fractures are most prevalent in:

    a.   adolescents.
    b.   elderly.
    c.   infants.
    d.   none of the above.

16. (b,1036)

16. ____ is the displacement of two bones in which the two bone surfaces partially lose contact.

    a.   Dislocation
    b.   Subluxation
    c.   Sublimation
    d.   Nonunion

17. (a,1036)

17. A tear in a ligament is commonly known as a:

    a.   sprain.
    b.   strain.
    c.   disunion.
    d   fracture.

18. (b,1036)

18. A tear in a tendon is commonly known as a:

a. sprain.
b. strain.
c. disunion.
d. fracture.

19. (a,1037)

19. _____ is the inflammation of tendon where it attaches to bone.

a. Epicondylitis
b. Endocondylitis
c. Bursitis
d. None of the above

20. (e,1038)

20. Following the Boston Marathon, seven runners were admitted to local hospitals with suspected myoglobinuria. This condition can also be seen following:

a. crush injuries.
b. fractures.
c. seizures.
d. a and b.
e. a, b, and c.

21. (d,1041)

21. All of the following may contribute to development of osteoporosis *except*:

a. parathyroid hormone dysfunction.
b. decreased estrogen levels.
c. heparin therapy.
d. increased intake of vitamin C.

22. (c,1043)

22. Mr. Ken Perry is a 56-year-old former computer programmer admitted to your hospital with a diagnosis of osteomalacia. From his history, you surmise all of the following to have contributed to the development of his osteomalacia except the fact that:

a. he takes anticonvulsants.
b. he underwent small bowel resection 3 years ago.
c. he has increased his intake of vitamin D.
d. he has pancreatic carcinoma.

23. (b,1045)

23. The cause of Paget disease is:

a. flouride deficiency
b. unknown at present
c. excess vitamin A
d. osteogenic sarcoma

24. (b,1043)

24. Although _____ is similar to osteomalacia, it occurs in growing bones of children.

a. Paget disease
b. rickets
c. osteomyelitis
d. none of the above

25. _____ is characterized by abnormal and excessive bone remodeling.

    a. Rickets
    b. Paget disease
    c. Osteoporosis
    d. Osteomyelitis

26. _____ may indicate that a bone tumor is malignant.

    a. An irregular nuclear border
    b. An increased nuclear-to-cytoplasmic ratio
    c. An excessive amount of chromatin
    d. Any of the above

27. The pattern of bone destruction indicative of an aggressive malignant tumor is:

    a. moth-eaten pattern.
    b. permeative pattern.
    c. geographic pattern.
    d. none of the above.

28. Kelly Akira is a 13-year-old female of Japanese heritage admitted to your hospital for evaluation and treatment of an osteosarcoma in her left distal femur. Which of the following is not true?

    a. Osteosarcomas always contain osteoid and callus, which is produced by anaplastic stromal cells.
    b. Ninety percent of osteosarcomas are located in the diaphysis of long bones.
    c. Initial symptoms are pain and swelling.
    d. Combined treatment is very effective.

29. A(n) _____ is a cartilage-forming tumor.

    a. chondrosarcoma
    b. adenoma
    c. hyalineoma
    d. each of the above

30. Bone tumors originate from:

    a. bone cells.
    b. cartilage.
    c. marrow.
    d. vascular tissue.
    e. all of the above

31. The chief pathological feature of degenerative joint disease is:

    a. degeneration and loss of the epiphyses.
    b. degeneration and loss of articular cartilage.
    c. degeneration and loss of synovial fluid.
    d. none of the above.

32. (d,1048) | 32. Noninflammatory joint disease is differentiated from inflammatory joint disease by all of the following *except*:

    a. the absence of synovial membrane inflammation.
    b. the lack of systemic signs and symptoms.
    c. normal synovial fluid.
    d. the presence or absence of pain and/or swelling.

33. (b,1050) | 33. Researchers have now determined that rheumatoid arthritis:

    a. develops most often in men.
    b. is an autoimmune disease.
    c. causes kyphosis.
    d. results in frequent fractures.

34. (c,1056) | 34. Peter Blackfoot is a 29-year-old Native American attorney recently diagnosed with ankylosing spondylitis. He is very interested in obtaining more information about his disease. Your patient teaching would include all of the following statements *except*:

    a. Diagnosis is made from history, physical examination, x-rays, and serum analysis for the presence of the histocompatibility antigen HLB-B27.
    b. Inflammation of the fibrocartilage in cartilaginous joints results in the erosion of bone structure, the organization of fibrous scar tissue, and eventual loss of joint mobility through fusion.
    c. The more common signs and symptoms of early disease include restricted spinal rotation and increased pain following physical activity.
    d. Usual treatment includes anti-inflammatory and analgesic medications, exercises, and physical therapy.

35. (a,1056) | 35. _____ is a chronic, inflammatory joint disease characterized by stiffening and fusion of the spine and sacroiliac joints.

    a. Ankylosing spondylitis
    b. Rheumatoid arthritis
    c. Paget disease
    d. Osteomyelitis

36. (a,1057) | 36. Which of the following people is at highest risk for the development of gout?

    a. men
    b. women
    c. children
    d. any of the above

37. (c,1057) | 37. Crystallization of _____ within the synovial fluid causes acute, painful inflammation of the joint, a condition known as gouty arthitis.

    a. purines
    b. pyrimidines
    c. uric acid
    d. acetic acid

38. (a,1058) | 38. A person diagnosed with gout is at risk for developing all of the following *except*:

    a. cholelithiasis.
    b. monoarticular arthritis.
    c. renal disease.
    d. deposits of tophi in and around the joints.

39. (a,1058)

39. The pathophysiology of gout is closely linked to:

   a. purine metabolism.
   b. pyrimidine metabolism.
   c. vitamin metabolism.
   d. amino acid metabolism.

40. (d,1058)

40. Clinical manifestations of gout may include:

   a. an increase in serum urate.
   b. recurrent attacks of monoarticular arthritis.
   c. renal disease.
   d. any of the above.

Matching

41. (c,1060)

41. ___ temporary or permanent muscle spasm or weakness

a. stess-induced muscle tension

42. (a,1060)

42. ___ muscle tension associated with anxiety

b. disuse atrophy

c. contracture

43. (b,1060)

43. ___ pathologic reduction in normal size muscle fibers after prolonged inactivity

d. myotonia

e. fibromyalgia

44. (d,1060)

44. ___ delayed relaxation after voluntary muscle contraction

45. (e,1060)

45. ___ chronic syndrome characterized by diffuse pain and tender points

Short Answer

46. McArdle disease is one of nine _____ diseases.

47. List the three causes of myositis.

48. List the three patterns of bone destruction caused by bone tumors.

49. About 50% of osteocarcomas occur _____.

50. What are the two types of myelogenic tumors?

Short Answers

46. Glycogen storage (1064)
47. Viral, bacterial, parasytic (1065)
48. Geographic pattern, moth-eaten pattern, permeative pattern (1067)
49. Around the knee area (1068)
50. Giant cell tumors, myelomas (1070)

Alterations of Musculoskeletal Function in Children

Name _____

True/False

1. (F,1075)   1. T   F   Musculoskeletal disorders in children are uncommon.

2. (F,1076)   2. T   F   The earliest pathologic changes in scoliosis occur in the vertebrae.

3. (T,1078)   3. T   F   Children are more prone to joint involvement with osteomyelitis.

4. (T,1084)   4. T   F   Between 60% and 80% of female carriers of Duchenne muscular dystrophy have elevated serum CK levels.

5. (F,1076)   5. T   F   Developmental displacement of the hip does not run in families and therefore is considered to be strictly an environmentally caused disease.

6. (T,1076)   6. T   F   Foot deformities in children are common and may be a result of intrauterine posi-tioning or true embryonic malformations.

7. (F,1076)   7. T   F   Lateral deviation of the foot away from the midline of the body is called adduc-tion.

8. (T,1076)   8. T   F   Idiopathic scoliosis is the most common form of scoliosis.

9. (F,1076)   9. T   F   Poor posture may result in structural scoliosis.

10. (T,1078)   10. T   F   Septic arthritis is frequently associated with osteomyelitis in newborns.

11. (F,1080)   11. T   F   In both adult and juvenile rheumatoid arthritis, the large joints are predominantly affected.

12. (F,1079)   12. T   F   Unlike adult-onset arthritis, juvenile rheumatoid arthritis is not a syndrome that is often accompanied by systemic manifestations.

13. (T,1082)   13. T   F   The onset of Duchenne muscular dystrophy usually occurs at three years of age.

14. (T,1083)   14. T   F   Limb girdle muscular dystrophy has a poorly defined mode of inheritance.

15. (F,1087)   15. T   F   Rhabdomyosarcomas originate in smooth muscle.

Multiple Choice

16. (d,1082)

16. Muscular dystrophy causes:

    a.   hypertrophy of smooth muscle cells.
    b.   degeneration of smooth muscle cells.
    c.   hypertrophy of striated muscle fibers.
    d.   degeneration of striated muscle fibers.

17. (b,1081)

17. Legg-Calvé-Perthes disease peaks at age:

    a.   3
    b.   6
    c.   9
    d.   12

18. (e,1081)

18. Possible causes of Legg-Calvé-Perthes disease are:

    a.   thyroid deficiency.
    b.   trauma.
    c.   infection.
    d.   a and c.
    e.   a, b, and c.

19. (c,1082)

19. Osgood-Schlatter disease affects the:

    a.   shoulder.
    b.   elbow.
    c.   knee.
    d.   hip.

20. (a,1080)

20. Treatment for children with juvenile rheumatoid arthritis is:

    a.   supportive.
    b.   curative.
    c.   nonexistent.
    d.   experimental.

21. (c,1076)

21. Clubfoot is:

    a.   metatarsus adductus.
    b.   metatarsus abductus.
    c.   talipes equinovarus.
    d.   none of the above.

22. (c,1076)

22. Osteogenesis imperfecta is also known as:

    a.   clubfoot.
    b.   Legg-Calvé-Perthes disease.
    c.   brittle bone disease.
    d.   rhabdosarcoma.

23. (e,1084)

23. Complications of Duchenne muscular dystrophy include:

    a. kyphoscoliosis.
    b. megacolon.
    c. mental retardation.
    d. a and c.
    e. a, b, and c.

24. (c,1076)

24. The major error in osteogenesis imperfecta lies in the synthesis of:

    a. elastin.
    b. glycoproteins.
    c. collagen.
    d. calcium salts.

25. (d,1085)

25. Seventy-five percent of children with Duchenne muscular dystrophy will die prior to age:

    a. 18
    b. 19
    c. 20
    d. 21

26. (e,1084)

26. Duchenne muscular dystrophy can be diagnosed:

    a. prenatally.
    b. at birth.
    c. during early childhood.
    d. a and b.
    e. a, b, and c.

27. (b,1076)

27. Structural scoliosis with no known cause, termed _____ scoliosis, accounts for at least 65% of the cases.

    a. etiopathic
    b. idiopathic
    c. iatrogenic
    d. none of the above

28. (a,1076)

28. Osteomyelitis may be defined as:

    a. inflammation of the bone and bone marrow.
    b. inflammation of the osteoblasts.
    c. inflammation of the osteocytes.
    d. inflammation of the osteoclasts.

29. (c,1081)

29. The three clinical stages of osteochondrosis include all of the following *except*:

    a. avascular necrosis.
    b. acute inflammation in tissues adjacent to areas of necrosis.
    c. bone marrow hypertrophy.
    d. healing and repair.

30. (a,1082)

30. The incidence of Osgood-Schlatter disease is greater in _____ than in _____:

    a. boys, girls
    b. girls, boys
    c. neither girls nor boys

31. (e,1082)

31. Classification of the muscular dystrophies is based on:

    a. age of onset.
    b. rate of progression.
    c. distribution of muscle involvement.
    d. inheritance patterns.
    e. all of the above.

32. (a,1082)

32. Which of the following muscular dystrophy syndromes demonstrates an X-linked recessive mode of inheritance?

    a. Duchenne dystrophy
    b. facioscapulohumeral dystrophy
    c. myotonic dystrophy
    d. a and b
    e. a, b, and c

33. (a,1083)

33. Classic Duchenne muscular dystrophy has a history of an _____ inheritance pattern.

    a. X-linked recessive
    b. X-linked dominant
    c. autosomal dominant
    d. autosomal recessive

34. (e,1085)

34. The most common childhood bone tumor is:

    a. fibrosarcoma.
    b. chondrosarcoma.
    c. non-Hodgkin lymphoma of the bone.
    d. Ewing sarcoma.
    e. osteosarcoma.

35. (c,1082)

35. _____ is present in normal muscle cells and absent in muscle cells of Duchenne muscular dystrophy muscle cells.

    a. Actin
    b. Myosin
    c. Dystrophin
    d. Troponin

36. (c,1087)

36. A major predictor of prognosis for Ewing sarcoma is:

    a. age of onset.
    b. size of tumor.
    c. presence of metastasis.
    d. gender of child.

37. (d,1085)

37. There is a link between osteosarcoma and:

    a. rhabdomyosarcoma.
    b. Ewing sarcoma.
    c. fibroma.
    d. retinoblastoma.

38. (d,1087)

38. The most common soft tissue tumor during childhood is:

 a. chondrosarcoma.
 b. fibrosarcoma.
 c. leiomyosarcoma.
 d. rhabdomyosarcoma.

39. (b,1085)

39. Osteosarcomas in children occur mainly in the _____ of long bones.

 a. epiphyses
 b. metaphyses
 c. marrow
 d. osteocytes

40. (a,1086)

40. _____ probably originates from cells within the bone marrow space and does not involve osteoblasts.

 a. Ewing sarcoma
 b. Leukemia
 c. Fibrosarcoma
 d. Lymphoma

41. (d,1087)

41. Rhabdosarcoma can develop anywhere _____ muscle is located.

 a. cardiac
 b. smooth
 c. involuntary
 d. striated

Matching

42. (c,1076)

42. ___ kidney bean-shaped foot   a. Legg-Calvé-Perthes disease

43. (d,1076)

43. ___ clubfoot   b. osteogenesis imferfecta

44. (a,1081)

44. ___ anatalgic abductor lurch   c. metatarsus adductus

45. (b,1076)

45. ___ brittle bone disease   d. talipes equinovarus

Short Answer

46. What are the names and causes of the two types of scoliosis?

47. Childhood osteomyelitis occur most often between ages _____ and _____.

48. What are the three modes of juvenile rheumatoid arthritis onset?

49. Osgood-Schlatter disease is tendinitis of:

50. What is the most common presenting complaint in osteosarcoma?

Short Answers

46. Nonstructural—results from a cause other than the spine itself
    Structural—curvature associated with vertebral rotation (1076)
47. 3 and 12 years (1076)
48. Pauciarticular, polyarthritis, and systemic disease (1080)
49. The anterior patellar tendon (1082)
50. Pain (1085)

Structure, Function, and Disorders of the Integument

Name _____

True/False

1. (F,1091)	1. T	F	The main function of the skin is temperature regulation.
2. (T,1092)	2. T	F	The dermis layer of skin is thicker than the epidermis.
3. (F,1093)	3. T	F	With aging, a person's skin becomes thicker.
4. (F,1102)	4. T	F	Psoriasis is an inflammatory skin condition.
5. (T,1092)	5. T	F	Dermal appendages include glands.
6. (F,1107)	6. T	F	Carbuncles are boils and not infected hair follicles.
7. (F,1107)	7. T	F	Cellulitis is a sterile inflammation caused by an autoimmune mechanism.
8. (T,1107)	8. T	F	Erysipelas is an acute infection of the skin most often caused by group *A streptococci*.
9. (T,1107)	9. T	F	Cytomegalovirus is a type of herpes virus.
10. (F,1107)	10. T	F	Impetigo is a superficial lesion caused by herpes simplex virus.
11. (T,1107)	11. T	F	Shingles and chicken pox are both caused by the same herpes virus.
12. (T,1108)	12. T	F	Warts are benign lesions of the skin caused by human papilloma virus.
13. (F,1114)	13. T	F	Melanoma is a malignant tumor of the skin originating from keratinocytes, the cells of the skin that synthesize the pigment melanin.

Multiple Choice

14. (d,1093)

14. Keratinocytes are found in which layer of the skin?

a. epidermis
b. dermis
c. hypodermis
d. all of the above

15. (e,1093) | 15. _____ may be found in the epidermis.

- a. Keratinocytes
- b. Melanocytes
- c. Langerhans cells
- d. a and b
- e. a, b, and c

16. (a,1093) | 16. _____ of the epidermis are involved in initiating the immune response.

- a. Langerhans cells
- b. Merkel cells
- c. Keratinocytes
- d. Melanocytes

17. (e,1092) | 17. Which of the following are structural units of nails?

- a. proximal nail fold
- b. matrix
- c. hyponychium
- d. nail plate
- e. all of the above

18. (a,1092) | 18. Growth of sebaceous glands is stimulated by _____, and their enlargement is one of the early signs of puberty.

- a. testosterone
- b. estrogen
- c. vitamin D
- d. progesterone

19. (b,1092) | 19. Of the sweat glands, the _____ glands are most abundant in the axilla and genital areas.

- a. eccrine
- b. apocrine
- c. sebaceous
- d. none of the above

20. (b,1093) | 20. More heat may be conserved by the body if blood is shunted away from the arteriovenous anastomoses in the:

- a. epidermis.
- b. dermis.
- c. hypodermis.
- d. a and c.
- e. a, b, and c.

Emily Moore, a 78-year-old widowed female, has been admitted to a surgical unit for treatment of a decubitus ulcer over her sacrum. Ms. Moore has been bedridden since having a CVA with right-sided hemiplegia 3 weeks prior to admission to this nursing unit. Ms. Moore appears confused at times but hears well and nods her head rather than speaking. She answers "yes" or "no" to most questions even though other answers would be more appropriate. Ms. Moore is accompanied to the unit by her daughter.

21. (d,1099)

21. A decubitus ulcer is most often caused by:

    a. arteriosclerosis.
    b. malnutrition.
    c. mental depression.
    d. unrelieved pressure.

22. (a,1100)

22. Sacral area decubiti commonly develop from shearing or friction forces that are:

    a. parallel to skin surfaces.
    b. perpendicular to skin surfaces.
    c. varying perpendicular and parallel forces.
    d. all of the above.

23. (a,1099)

23. The first indication of a beginning pressure area is:

    a. redness.
    b. whiteness.
    c. blueness.
    d. no color change.

24. (c,1100)

24. Initial turning schedules for Ms. Moore include turning her every:

    a. 30 min (1/2 hr).
    b. 60 min (1 hr).
    c. 120 min (2 hr).
    d. 240 min (4 hr).

25. (b,1100)

25. Dressings applied to Ms. Moore's decubitus should be:

    a. flat and dry.
    b. flat and moist.
    c. bulky and dry.
    d. bulky and moist.

26. (d,1107-
    1108)

26. Chicken pox may be followed years later by:

    a. erysipelas.
    b. poliomyelitis.
    c. warts (verrucae).
    d. herpes zoster.

27. (d,1100)

27. _____ are more prone to developing keloids.

    a. Blacks
    b. Whites
    c. Orientals
    d. a and c
    e. a, b, and c

28. (b,1100)

28. Keloids are sharply elevated, irregularly shaped, progressively enlarging scars caused by excessive amounts of _____ in the corneum during connective tissue repair.

  a. elastin
  b. collagen
  c. stroma
  d. reticular fibers

29. (e,1100)

29. Pruritus is a symptom that may be associated with:

  a. lice.
  b. eczema.
  c. cholestatic liver disease.
  d. renal failure.
  e. any of the above.

30. (a,1101)

30. _____ is an inflammatory response of the skin caused by endogenous and exogenous agents and is often considered synonymous with dermatitis.

  a. Eczema
  b. Psoriasis
  c. Atopic dermatitis
  d. None of the above

31. (d,1102)

31. Seborrheic dermatitis is a common chronic inflammation of the skin involving the:

  a. scalp.
  b. nasolabial folds.
  c. axillae.
  d. all of the above.

32. (e,1102)

32. The mode of inheritance of psoriasis is clearly by an:

  a. autosomal dominant gene.
  b. autosomal recessive gene.
  c. X-linked dominant gene.
  d. X-linked recessive gene.
  e. HLA-associated mode.

33. (b,1103)

33. The etiologic agent of pityriasis rosea is a(n):

  a. X-linked gene.
  b. virus.
  c. bacteria.
  d. none of the above.

34. (b,1104)

34. Acne vulgaris is an inflammatory disorder of the:

  a. apocrine glands.
  b. pilosebaceous follicle.
  c. hair follicle.
  d. eccrine gland.
  e. all of the above.

35. (d,1106)

35. Which of the listed dermatologic conditions causes formation of erythematose bullous lesions?

    a. pemphigus
    b. acne vulgaris
    c. systemic lupus erythematosus
    d. Stevens-Johnson syndrome

36. (c,1105)

36. _____ is an autoimmune disease.

    a. Stasis dermatitis
    b. Tinea infection
    c. Systemic lupus erythematosus
    d. Folliculitis

37. (b,1107)

37. _____ is a chronic blister-forming disease of the skin and oral mucous membranes.

    a. Systemic lupus erythematosus
    b. Pemphigus
    c. Psoriasis
    d. Eczema

38. (b,1108)

38. _____ are a collection of infected hair follicles.

    a. Furuncles
    b. Carbuncles
    c. Erysipelas
    d. Folliculitis

39. (b,1108)

39. Tinea corporis (ringworm) is a _____ infection of the skin.

    a. nematode
    b. fungal
    c. viral
    d. bacterial

40. (d,1109)

40. Candidiasis is likely to be exacerbated by:

    a. Cushing disease.
    b. diabetes mellitus.
    c. systemic antibiotics.
    d. all of the above.

41. (b,1111)

41. In scleroderma, 50% of patients die within _____ years of onset.

    a. 1
    b. 5
    c. 10
    d. 15

42. (d,1112)

42. Which malignant skin lesion is the most serious?

    a. basal cell carcinoma
    b. squamous cell carcinoma
    c. Kaposi sarcoma
    d. malignant melanoma

43. (a,1118)

43. Hypovolemic shock in persons with severe burns is a result of:

   a.   increased capillary permeability.
   b.   elevation of hematocrit.
   c.   extravasation of fluids.
   d.   decreased peripheral resistance.

44. (c,1118)

44. The fluid of choice for fluid volume replacement in persons with severe burns is:

   a.   normal saline.
   b.   fresh frozen plasma.
   c.   Ringer's lactate.
   d.   albumin.

45. (c,1121)

45. Excessive growth of hair is referred to as:

   a.   alopecia.
   b.   psoriasis.
   c.   hirsutism.
   d.   pruritus.

Matching

46. (h,1094)   46. ___   macule   a. elevated, firm lesion less than 1 cm in diameter

47. (c,1095)   47. ___   nodule   b. solid or fluid-filled elevated lesion

48. (b,1095)   48. ___   cyst   c. elevated, firm, circumscribed dermal lesion

49. (a,1094)   49. ___   papule   d. elevated, firm, rough lesion larger than 1 cm

50. (e,1096)   50. ___   bulla   e. large vesicle

51. (d,1094)   51. ___   plaque   f. elevated, irregular-shaped edematous area

52. (g,1096)   52. ___   telangiectasia   g. fine, irregular red lines

53. (f,1095)   53. ___   wheal   h. flat, circumscribed color change of less than 1 cm in diameter

Short Answer

54. What percentage of body weight is accounted for by the skin?

55. Why does aging skin wrinkle?

56. List the four types of pemphigus.

57. What type of lesions are most commonly associated with type 1 hypersensitivity reactions?

58. List two diseases transmitted by ticks.

59. List the three phases of keratoacanthoma.

60. What are the three essential elements of survival of major burn injury?

Short Answers

54. About 20% (1091)
55. Loss of elastin with aging produces wrinkles (1093)
56. Pemphigus vulgaris, pemphigus foliaceus, pemphigus erythematosus, paraneoplastic pemphigus (1105-1106)
57. Urticarial lesions (1110)
58. Rocky mountain spotted fever, tularemia, lyme disease (1111)
59. Proliferative stage, mature stage, involution stage (1112)
60. Meticulous wound management, adequate fluids and nutrition, early surgical excision and grafting (1120)

Alterations of the Integument in Children

Name _____

True/False

1. (F,1129)	1. T F	Impetigo is a common viral skin infection in infants and children.
2. (T,1128)	2. T F	Atopic dermatitis is the most common cause of eczema in children.
3. (T,1130)	3. T F	Staphylococcal scaled-skin syndrome is more common in children than in adults.
4. (F,1130)	4. T F	Scalded skin syndrome is the result of a staphylococcal infection of burned skin.
5. (F,1130)	5. T F	In cases of of staphylococcal scalded skin syndrome, the most effective treatment is direct application of antibiotics to the skin.
6. (T,1130)	6. T F	Fungal disorders of the skin are known as tinea.
7. (T,1130)	7. T F	The most common fungal infection in children is tinea capitis.
8. (F,1130)	8. T F	Tinea capitis, a fungal infection of the scalp, is the most common fungal infection of childhood and occurs most commonly in infants.
9. (T,1131)	9. T F	The distribution of molluscum contagiosum lesions in children is mainly on the trunk, face, and extremities.
10. (F,1133)	10. T F	Koplik spots are characteristic of rubella.
11. (T,1132)	11. T F	Pregnant women who contract rubella during the first trimester may have a fetus with congenital defects.
12. (T,1134)	12. T F	The varicella-zoster virus produces both chicken pox and herpes zoster.
13. (T,1134)	13. T F	Due to mass immunization, the world is virtually free of small pox.
14. (T,1134)	14. T F	Scabies is a contagious disease caused by the itch mite.
15. (F,1134)	15. T F	Scabies is an infectious disease caused by a herpes virus.
16. (T,1137)	16. T F	Nevus flammeus is a vascular disorder of the skin.
17. (F,1136)	17. T F	The majority of strawberry hemangiomas require surgical treatment.
18. (T,1137)	18. T F	Congenital malformation of the dermal capillaries is called portwine stain.

19. (F,1137)

19. T   F   Closure of sebaceous glands results in a dermatosis called miliara.

Multiple Choice

20. (d,1129)

20. Atopic dermatitis has a constellation of clinical features that include all of the following *except*:

a. severe pruritis.
b. chronic course.
c. appearance of age-dependent distribution of skin lesions.
d. infrequent exacerbations.

21. (c,1128)

21. Which of the following immunoglobulins is elevated in atopic dermatitis?

a. IgD
b. IgM
c. IgE
d. IgG

22. (c,1129)

22. Frequently, diaper dermatitis is secondarily infected with:

a. *E. coli.*
b. *Proteus.*
c. *Candida albicans.*
d. *Staphylococci.*

23. (b,1130)

23. Which type of impetigo is caused by streptococci infections?

a. bullous impetigo
b. vesicular impetigo
c. a and b
d. neither a nor b

24. (a,1130)

24. Bullous impetigo is caused by a strain of _____ that produces an exfoliative toxin which causes disruption in cellular adhesion.

a. *Staphylococcus aureus*
b. *Streptococcus*
c. *E. coli*
d. *Candida albicans*

25. (c,1130)

25. The etiologic agent of vesicular impetigo is:

a. *Staphylococcus aureus.*
b. *Candida albicans.*
c. *Streptococcus pyogenes.*
d. *Trichophyton tonsurans.*

26. (a,1129)

26. Most skin infections are:

a. superficial.
b. systemic.
c. life-threatening.
d. b and c.

27. (d,1131) | 27. A common source for the etiologic agent for tinea corporis is:

  a. young kittens
  b. young puppies
  c. hamsters
  d. a and b
  e. a, b, and c

28. (b,1131) | 28. _____ is also referred to as ringworm.

  a. Platyhelminthes
  b. Tinea corporis
  c. Thrush
  d. Psoriasis

29. (b,1131) | 29. The etiologic agent of molluscum contagiosum is:

  a. a bacteria.
  b. a virus.
  c. a fungus.
  d. a herpes virus.

30. (c,1131) | 30. Thrush is a superficial infection that commonly occurs in children and is caused by:

  a. *E. coli.*
  b. *Streptococci.*
  c. *Candida albicans.*
  d. *Staphylococci.*

31. (a,1131) | 31. Thrush may be defined as:

  a. the presence of *Candida* in the mucous membranes of the mouth of infants.
  b. the presence of bacteria in the nasal mucous membranes of infants.
  c. any viral infection of the mucous membranes of the mouth of infants.
  d. an acute immune response to oral medication, located in the mucosal lining of the mouth of infants.

32. (b,1132) | 32. Which of the following viral diseases has an incubation period of 14-21 days and a duration of 1-3 days?

  a. rubeola
  b. rubella
  c. roseola
  d. varicella

33. (a,1132) | 33. Rubella (German or three-day measles) is a common communicable disease of children caused by:

  a. a virus.
  b. a bacteria.
  c. a fungus.
  d. yeast.

34. (b,1132)   34. MMR vaccine should be administered after 15 months of age because:

      a.   children under this age are not susceptible to rubella.
      b.   by this time maternally acquired passive immunity has been depleted.
      c.   children under 15 months of age are more likely to have an allergic reaction to the vaccine.
      d.   none of the above.

35. (d,1132)   35. Rubeola is a highly contagious, acute _____ disease of children.

      a.   bacterial
      b.   fungal
      c.   nematode
      d.   viral

36. (b,1133)   36. The etiologic agent of chicken pox is:

      a.   a poxvirus.
      b.   a herpes virus.
      c.   adenovirus.
      d.   human papilloma virus.

37. (a,1134)   37. A fetus is most likely to be malformed if the mother contracts chicken pox during the _____ trimester of pregnancy.

      a.   first
      b.   second
      c.   third
      d.   any of the above

38. (b,1134)   38. The etiologic agent of smallpox is:

      a.   herpes virus.
      b.   poxvirus.
      c.   insects.
      d.   mites.

39. (e,1135)   39. All of the following are vascular disorders of the integument *except*:

      a.   strawberry hemiangioma.
      b.   cavernous hemiangioma.
      c.   nevus inflammeus.
      d.   salmon patches.
      e.   pediculosis.

Matching

40. (d,1134)   40. ____ scabies   a. fleas

41. (b,1135)   41. ____ pediculosis   b. lice infestation

42. (e,1136)   42. ____ 3- to 5-mm long, reddish brown bug   c. milaria

43. (a,1135)   43. ____ bite cats, dogs, and humans   d. itch mite

44. (c,1137)   44. ____ prolonged exposure to perspiration obstructs eccrine ducts   e. bed bug

Short Answer

45. List the three principal causative factors of acne vulgaris.

46. From 75% to 80% of individuals with atopic dermatitis have a personal or family history of what two diseases?

47. From what serious illness must staphylococcal scalded-skin syndrome be differentiated?

48. What type of virus is contained in measles vaccine?

49. What adult disease is a reactivation of the chickenpox virus?

50. List the three known types of louse that infest humans.

Short Answers

45. Abnormal keratinization of the follicular epithelium, excessive sebum production, proliferation of *Propionibacterium acnes* (1128)
46. Asthma, allergic rhinitis (hay fever) (1128)
47. Toxic epidermal necrosis (1130)
48. Live, attenuated virus (1133)
49. Herpes zoster (shingles) (1134)
50. The head louse, the body louse, and the crab or pubic louse (1135)